For my family, Joanna, Liam, Niall, Louie and Martin, with whom I now hope to spend more time. And for Hunter, whose advice about how to write I have endeavoured to follow over many years.

Concordance in Medical Consultations

A critical review

Kristian Pollock

Senior Research Fellow
School of Nursing
The University of Nottingham

Radcliffe Publishing
Oxford • Seattle

Radcliffe Publishing Ltd
18 Marcham Road
Abingdon
Oxon OX14 1AA
United Kingdom

www.radcliffe-oxford.com
Electronic catalogue and worldwide online ordering facility.

British Library Cataloguing in Publication Data

A catalogue record for this book is available from the British Library.

ISBN-10 1 85775 841 2
ISBN-13 978 1 85775 841 2

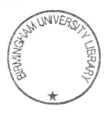

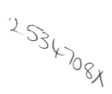

Typeset by Anne Joshua & Associates, Oxford
Printed and bound by TJ International Ltd, Padstow, Cornwall

Contents

Preface

Concordance is a recent addition to a clutch of topical constructs (including 'shared decision making', patient 'participation', 'satisfaction', 'choice', 'self-management' and 'patient expertise') which reflect the current academic and policy commitment to move away from the traditional paternalism of professional medicine towards a health service that is responsive to, and firmly centred on, patient preferences and assessment of care. The concept of concordance was first elaborated in the report *From Compliance to Concordance*, published by the Royal Pharmaceutical Society of Great Britain in 1997. It developed from a concern with the very high rate of patient non-compliance with prescribed medication, and a desire to find ways to reduce this. It involved movement from a focus on the perplexing irrationality of patients in failing to follow medical advice, to an understanding of the *reasonableness* of such actions when viewed from the patient perspective. Concordance places professional awareness of patients' knowledge and concerns about illness at the centre of effective consultations. It also acknowledges that, under all ordinary circumstances, patient preferences regarding treatment should be accorded priority over those of professionals. This is partly a pragmatic response to the reality of medicines use: regardless of what has been advised and prescribed, it is the patient who finally decides whether to take the medicines or not. In addition, concordance involves a recognition that patients' decisions about healthcare are based on values and goals that differ from, and may directly conflict with, those of clinical rationality. In an age of consumerism personal autonomy and self-determination are constituted as core attributes of citizenship. The appropriation of personal (patient) choice through the benign paternalism of traditional medicine is no longer regarded as acceptable. The application of concordance *should* have far-reaching consequences for clinical practice and the relationships between patients and health professionals.

My interest in concordance developed while I was joint holder (with Janet Grime at Keele University) of the Concordance Research Fellowship between 1999 and 2004. The Fellowship was awarded by the Royal Pharmaceutical Society and funded by the Department of Health. My research interests had always been in the area of lay perspectives of health and illness. During the Fellowship these were extended through a series of studies in which we explored patient and GP understandings of the diagnosis and treatment of depression in general practice, barriers to meeting the information needs of patients on acute psychiatric wards, and mental health service users' experience of complexity of healthcare provision in community settings. Our findings supported those of many other empirical studies which point to the *lack* of change in the bureaucratic format of medical consultations and the continuation of the passive and deferential role adopted by patients in interactions with health professionals. Despite decades of pressure for change, and a sustained rhetoric of patient-centred medicine, patients remain largely intimidated and mystified by complex bureaucratic systems of care and frequently disappointed by their superficial and perfunctory consultations with health professionals.

The capacity of professional medicine to resist change – and also concordance – is impressive, but perplexing. It is one of the issues I seek to address in this book. I suggest that a preoccupation with trying to change the relationship between the professional–patient dyad has deflected attention from the extent to which such relations are embedded in, and constrained by, wider administrative and organisational structures, especially as these relate to the operation of professional hierarchies and interprofessional deference and allegiances. Barriers to change also result from the inertia of a system which has evolved a highly stylised etiquette as an adaptive mechanism to contain the difficulties and tensions intrinsic to the medical consultation. Its therapeutic purpose and potential are often subordinate to the goal of achieving success as a *social* encounter.

The principles of concordance are deeply challenging to traditional professional roles and status. However, medicine has always displayed an ability to block change through tactics of appropriation and incorporation. Professionals have often shown particular difficulty giving up their monopoly of 'expertise' and in acknowledging the legitimacy of the patient perspective. Although the term 'concordance' has become quite widely used, its meaning is usually subverted by its employment as a synonym for 'compliance', albeit 'informed' compliance. A slightly more sophisticated version values professional elicitation of the patient perspective in order to more accurately tailor information as a means of overcoming the unhelpful *mis*conceptions that impede compliance. The original emphasis on the consultation as a negotiated *exchange*, in which the professional has something of value to learn from the patient, has largely been lost. The rhetoric of modernity and change provides an effective mask for inertia and conservatism.

As it has been applied and developed beyond the formulation of the original working party report, concordance has become practically equated with patient education, and the state of being 'fully informed'. Fully informed patients are assumed to be willing and able to make appropriate ('correct') decisions about treatment and assume greater responsibility for healthcare. Information is usually regarded as fundamentally and self-evidently a good thing, and an important lever for increasing the 'patient centredness' of healthcare. However, I argue that although information may be often desired and positive in its effects, it is not always or necessarily so. Information may be conflicting and confusing, and a source of increased uncertainty rather than a means of reducing anxiety. Knowledge is not always benign and may be burdensome: an obligation, rather than an entitlement. There is considerable and accumulating evidence that patients' desire for information is much more variable and equivocal than is generally assumed. The current enthusiasm for educating patients is running ahead of the research evidence, revealing a strong underlying ideological motivation. This is an important topic which requires much further attention and investigation.

Finally, I suggest that the most neglected factor impeding the development of patient-centred medicine is a considerable and persisting conservatism on the part of patients themselves. It is not at all clear that many, far less all, patients actively want to sign up as reflexive consumers of healthcare. Much more needs to be known about people's comfort with the extended responsibilities of the 'expert patient' role. Considerable benefits may be gained from a degree of medical paternalism, and costs incurred in patients' assumption of greater responsibility for healthcare. There is, however, plenty of evidence, which goes back many years, about what patients positively value in medical encounters. This includes establishing good relationships with health professionals, the feeling of being listened to and reassured, that concerns have been acknowledged and understood, and being treated with courtesy and respect. It is not so much the information that is conveyed as the understanding that is negotiated that is important in determining patients' 'satisfaction' with medical consultations. There is nothing new or revelatory about this list of attributes, but they are as far away from being routinely implemented now as they were when the first accounts of the patient perspective were written in the middle decades of the last century.

The ideals of concordance (in its original form) may be exemplary, but it is not clear to what extent they resonate with the concerns and issues which most patients find most pressing. Current policy is framed in terms of assumptions about what patients want or *should* regard as desirable (e.g. the specious propaganda relating to 'choosing health'), but which are not borne out by a careful review of the evidence. A truly patient-centred – and concordant – medical practice needs to start from a genuine professional awareness and understanding of the patient perspective. In particular, it should acknowledge the central importance of attending to the patient's *experience* of illness as an arbitrary and capricious manifestation of misfortune, rather than an occasion for the attribution of blame and personal irresponsibility. Only then will there be a chance for the reorientation of the professional preoccupation with non-compliance as a technical problem of defective patient behaviour towards an acceptance of the radical shift in underlying philosophy and culture that is required for the development of a genuinely concordant medical practice.

Kristian Pollock
September 2005

About the author

Kristian Pollock is a senior research fellow in the School of Nursing at Nottingham University. She studied social anthropology at the Universities of Edinburgh and Cambridge and has carried out qualitative research in a range of health service settings. She has a particular interest in lay and professional constructions of illness and health, the social and personal significance of medicines, 'knowledge' as a resource in coping with illness and professional–patient interaction in medical consultations. Her interest in concordance developed during the course of a five-year Concordance Research Fellowship, funded by the Department of Health, which she held jointly with Janet Grime at the Department of Medicines Management at Keele University.

Acknowledgements

Thanks are due to those organisations that have kindly given permission for reproduction of copyrighted material. Although we have tried to trace and contact all copyright holders before publication, this has not been possible in every case. If notified, the publisher will be pleased to make any necessary arrangements at the earliest opportunity.

Chapter One

Introduction

Within the field of healthcare the terms 'compliance' and 'non-compliance' refer to the extent to which patients follow (or not) the regimens recommended by their doctors. An enormous amount of research over several decades has shown consistently that between one third and one half of patients do not follow their doctors' advice and in particular fail to take the medicines prescribed for them (Carter, Taylor & Levenson 2003; Donovan 1995; Donovan & Blake 1992; Haynes & Sackett 1979; Sackett & Haynes 1976; Stimson 1974; Trostle 1998). The manifest failure of so many patients to act in their own best interests has baffled the medical establishment. No distinctive characteristics of non-compliant individuals have been established, and the range of illnesses eliciting non-compliant behaviour runs across the spectrum from trivial to life-threatening. In one study Rovelli *et al.* found that patient non-compliance with immunosuppressive drugs following organ transplant caused a higher incidence of graft loss than uncontrollable rejection affecting patients who had adhered to treatment as prescribed. Eighteen per cent of renal transplant patients were found to be non-compliant with treatment and the majority (91%) of these subsequently experienced either organ rejection or death. The comparable failure rate for compliant patients was 18% (Rovelli *et al.* 1989). The high rates of 'non-compliance' among AIDS patients have also been well established (Chesney, Morin & Sherr 2002; Wright 2000). Thousands of studies of non-compliance and how to modify patient behaviour have been conducted over the last three decades. However, this enormous effort has made no discernible impact on the consistently high rates of reported non-adherence. The mismatch between medical prescription and patient behaviour has persisted, and manifests itself in many different forms (Box 1.1).

Box 1.1 Some types of 'non-compliant' behaviour

- Not taking a prescribed medicine
- Taking a higher dose of the medicine than was prescribed
- Taking less than the prescribed dose
- Taking the medicine more often than prescribed
- Taking the medicine less often than prescribed
- Taking 'drug holidays' from time to time
- Modifying treatment to accommodate other activities, such as work and social activities (e.g. missing a dose before social drinking)
- Stopping the medicine without finishing the course
- Not getting the prescription made up
- Taking additional medicines (Over the counter (OTC) or Prescription only medicines (POM))

- Continuing with behaviours (e.g. relating to diet, alcohol, smoking) against medical advice
- A combination of any of the above

Non-compliance clearly has enormous significance for the healthcare system. As health policy is increasingly driven by cost containment strategies attention has focused on the need to reduce wasted and inappropriate expenditure. The widespread failure of many patients to take their medicines as prescribed – or even at all – constitutes a huge squandering of effort and resources. It subverts the aim of professional treatment and is also a major source of suboptimal health outcomes. In a climate of medical practice dominated by the principles and self-evident rationality of Evidence-Based Medicine, the failure of large numbers of patients to take prescribed medicines appears both inexplicable and intolerable.

In 1995 the Royal Pharmaceutical Society of Great Britain undertook an investigation of non-compliance, with a view to developing practical recommendations for improving medicine taking among patients. This inquiry led in an unanticipated direction, and resulted in the usefulness of the concept of compliance being seriously questioned. In 1997 it published a report, *From Compliance to Concordance*, in which the concept of 'concordance' was advocated as a tool for radically changing the culture of prescribing and the substance of the relationship between health professionals and patients (RPSGB 1997). The members of the working party had consulted widely in the course of their investigations. However, in developing the concept of concordance, the discussions that were held with groups of patients and patient representatives were held to be particularly significant (Marinker 1997; Marinker 2004).

Concordance opens up the problem of non-compliance by explicitly recognising and valuing the patient perspective in medicine taking, rather than confining consideration of the issue to a narrow focus on medical values and rationality. Successful medicine taking rests on an agreement between professional and patient, and a mutual understanding of the different concerns and goals of treatment. The competence of the patient is acknowledged, along with the legitimacy of his beliefs and preferences in relation to healthcare, even where these differ from those of the professional. Ideally, differences between these perspectives would be resolved through negotiated consensus. However, it is accepted that, in all ordinary circumstances, the final decision about treatment rests with the patient.

The outcome of a concordant consultation may be that patient and practitioner disagree about the best course of action. A concordant consultation does not mean that the health professional is under any obligation to practise 'bad medicine', or accede to requests from patients that he considers to be unreasonable or inappropriate. In an ideal encounter, however, both parties would be aware of, and able to understand, the other's reasons for adhering to a different position, and perhaps be able to achieve a degree of compromise or negotiated consensus. In the common scenario where there is a range of options to be considered, there is scope for patient choice of treatment. Where patients are encouraged to state their preferences, and to actively participate in the process of decision making about illness management, it is assumed that they are more likely to be committed to the treatment which follows from this. Accepting the patient's choice of treatment, even though this may not be the preferred option from the professional point of view, may produce a better therapeutic gain if it results in treatment being accepted rather than rejected. The prescription of medicines which are unwanted or unused should be substantially reduced, with a consequent reduction in avoidable cost. Equally as significant, patients' experience of medical encounters and the quality of service provision should be improved. In the concordant model, this is taken to be a valid outcome of healthcare.

Concordance can be regarded as an extension of the principles of patient-centred medicine, particularly as these are applied to the activities of medicine taking and prescribing. Patient-centred medicine is central to the articulation of government health policy (Department of Health 1991, 1996, 1999, 2000, 2001, 2002). A more responsive and user-driven service is seen as a means to the development of a more cost-effective, socially accountable and higher quality health service. The emphasis on the satisfaction of individual needs and aspirations accords with the primacy of individual autonomy as a value within the system of corporate industrialism of the modern state. Concordance, like compliance, has a social history. The following chapters trace the development of both concepts, in the context of the major influences exerted from outside medicine as well as within it, before making an assessment of the present and future contribution of concordance to the practice of healthcare.

References

Carter S, Taylor D and Levenson R (2003) *A Question of Choice – compliance in medicine taking: a preliminary review*. Medicines Partnership, London.

Chesney MA, Morin M and Sherr L (2002) Adherence to HIV combination therapy. *Social Science and Medicine*. **50**: 1599–1605.

Department of Health (1991) *The Patient's Charter*. Department of Health, London.

Department of Health (1996) *Patient Partnership: building a collaborative strategy*. Department of Health, National Health Service Executive, London.

Department of Health (1999) *Patient and Public Involvement in the New NHS*. Department of Health, London.

Department of Health (2000) *The NHS Plan: a plan for investment, a plan for reform*. Department of Health, London.

Department of Health (2001) *The Expert Patient: a new approach to chronic disease management for the 21st century*. Department of Health, London.

Department of Health (2002) *Learning from Bristol: the DH response to the report of the public inquiry into children's heart surgery at the Bristol Royal Infirmary 1984–1995*. Department of Health, London.

Donovan J (1995) Patient decision making: the missing ingredient in compliance research. *International Journal of Technology Assessment in Health Care*. **11**: 443–55.

Donovan J and Blake D (1992) Patient non-compliance: deviance or reasoned decision-making? *Social Science and Medicine*. **35**(5): 507–13.

Haynes RB and Sackett DL (1979) *Compliance in Health Care*. Johns Hopkins University Press, Baltimore.

Marinker M (1997) Writing prescriptions is easy. *BMJ*. **314**: 747–8.

Marinker M (2004) From compliance to concordance: a personal view. In: C Bond (ed.) *Concordance: a partnership in medicine-taking*. Pharmaceutical Press, London, pp. 1–7.

Rovelli M, Palmeri D, Vossler E, Bartus S, Hull D and Schweizer R (1989) Noncompliance in organ transplant patients. *Transplantation Proceedings.* **21**(1): 833–4.

RPSGB (1997) *From Compliance to Concordance: achieving shared goals in medicine taking.* RPSGB, London.

Sackett DL and Haynes R (1976) *Compliance with Therapeutic Regimes.* Johns Hopkins University Press, Baltimore.

Stimson G (1974) Obeying doctor's orders: a view from the other side. *Social Science and Medicine.* **8**: 97–104.

Trostle JA (1998) Medical compliance as an ideology. *Social Science and Medicine.* **27**: 1299–308.

Wright M (2000) The old problem of adherence: research on treatment adherence and its relevance for HIV/AIDS. *Aids Care.* **12**: 703–10.

Chapter Two

The medical construction of compliance

The failure of patients to take medicines as prescribed by their physician appears to be longstanding. Hippocrates is reported to have cautioned physicians against accepting the accuracy of patients' reported compliance (Trostle 1988: 1300). There is evidence that professional concern with non-compliance predates the mid-twentieth century development of a truly effective pharmacopoeia. From the mid-nineteenth century, medical concern over control of patient behaviour and medicine taking was bound up with the consolidation of professional authority and the development of commercial interests and predated the discovery of effective treatments (Freidson 1970; Schwartz, Soumeris & Ajorn 1989; Trostle 1998). In the early decades of the twentieth century, the profession successfully appropriated control over access to infant feeding formula and nutritional supplements and the information given to mothers about how to use it. This illustrates the growing concern of doctors to influence the health-related behaviours of the lay population, and acquire control over access to information. It was also an early instance of the development of compliance as a marketing device by the pharmaceutical companies (Trostle 1998). Lerner (1997) describes the censorious medical response to TB patients after the First World War who failed to cooperate with what treatment was available, and discharged themselves prematurely from hospital in large numbers. However, the availability from the 1940s of the sulphonamides and antibiotics, and thereafter an increasingly large range of very effective treatments, substantially boosted medical authority and focused attention on the irrational and vexatious nature of non-compliance among patients. It was apparent early on that even with these new, very effective (and expensive) treatments patients often failed to complete their prescribed course of treatment. This behaviour was consistent across all social strata. Patients now came to be regarded as 'disobedient' rather than ethnically or socially degraded, as had formerly been the case with non-compliant TB sufferers (Lerner 1997).

The terms 'compliance' and 'non-compliance' were in use from the 1960s, but really became established with the work of Sackett and Haynes and their colleagues in the mid-1970s (Haynes & Sackett 1979; Sackett & Haynes 1976). These early compliance researchers documented the extent of patient non-adherence to medicine taking and sought to explain it. However, the range and sensitivity of their analysis and conclusions has been buried under the simplistic message that up to half of patients do not take their medicines as prescribed, and the associated assumptions about patient incompetence and irrationality that have become firmly entrenched within professional medical culture.

A distinction has been made between intentional and non-intentional non-compliance. The latter results from patient failure to follow instructions about treatment because these are in some way inadequate to enable a clear and accurate understanding of what is required, or practical and physical difficulties make it difficult for patients to do so. Compliance research has directed most attention to investigating and explaining intentional non-compliance, where patients deliberately alter their prescribed treatment regimes. However, early researchers in this area were sensitive to the problem and extent of non-intentional non-compliance, and understood that the remedy lay largely with health service providers rather than patients. They acknowledged the considerable reduction that could be achieved through straightforward changes to prescribing information and labels, simplification of medication regimes and modifications to administrative routines and processes regulating and facilitating patient access to healthcare services. Simple measures such as shortening waiting times for appointments or sending reminder calls or letters were found to improve figures for patient consultation and clinic attendance (Canada 1976; Fitzgerald 1976; Gibson 1979; Gordis 1979; Haynes 1976a; Ley 1982; McGavock *et al.* 1993; McKenney 1979; Sackett 1976).

Effective strategies to reduce intentional non-compliance have been more difficult to find. No association between specific patient characteristics and compliance behaviour has been established (Haynes 1976a). This is true also of the (non-)relationship between patient knowledge and information and compliance (Carter, Taylor & Levenson 2003; Gray, Wykes & Gournay 2002; Haynes 1976b; MacPherson, Jerrom & Hughes 1996) and despite the huge amount of effort that has been invested over several decades into trying to correct the information deficit that is assumed to underly much non-adherent behaviour. Early compliance work, however, was often sensitive to the importance of patient values, patient defined outcomes, partnership between patients and professionals and the need to tailor treatment regimes to individual goals and preferences (Haynes & Sackett 1979; Sackett & Haynes 1976). For example, Gordis (1979) suggested that compliance was only one among many factors determining health outcomes. Hogue (1979) emphasised the need to acknowledge the patient perspective, and that this might differ from professional objectives. Jonsen (1979) also recognised that patients may hold and even prioritise a number of legitimate goals as well as health.

Compliance researchers have always been motivated by a desire to optimise the health gain to be derived from taking medicines, and have seen non-adherence to be a major obstacle in achieving this. However, from the outset Haynes and Sackett cautioned that patients did not always benefit from treatment or healthcare or even from taking their medicines as prescribed (Haynes & Sackett 1979; Sackett & Haynes 1976). The iatrogenic effects of treatment might outweigh the benefits, and not all prescribed medicines were appropriate or effective. More subtle disadvantages could flow from medical diagnosis and intervention where this served to undermine people's confidence in their health, provoked debilitating anxiety about illness or generated a degree of adverse labelling and social stigma. For example, in one of his studies, Haynes recorded an increased amount of absenteeism from work among people diagnosed with hypertension especially those who were less compliant with treatment (Haynes 1979).

Haynes and Sackett (Haynes & Sackett 1979; Sackett 1976; Sackett & Haynes 1976) stipulated that compliance was only a reasonable or appropriate patient response if three basic criteria were met:

1 the diagnosis should be correct
2 treatment should be effective and appropriate
3 the patient had given informed consent.

These conditions are frequently problematic, however, and often not realised in practice. Patient dissatisfaction with treatment information, and the inadequacy of much of the information that is available to them are longstanding complaints (Coulter, Entwistle & Gilbert 1998; Coulter, Entwistle & Gilbert 1999; Dixon-Woods 2001; Ley 1997). These issues are taken up in Chapter 8. Growing awareness of the uncertainty of medical diagnosis and the variable and untested nature of most interventions and treatment from the 1970s onward (Cochrane 1995) was a spur to the development of Evidence-Based Medicine (EBM) which has been a dominant force in medical thought (if not practice) over the past two decades, and is taken up for consideration in the following chapter. As with compliance research, the movement to EBM was also spearheaded by Sackett and Haynes (Haynes & Haines 1998; Haynes, Devereaux & Guyatt 2002; Sackett *et al.* 1996; Sackett *et al.* 1997).

It is worth noting that it is not just patients who fail to follow medical advice and guidelines for good practice. The significance and extent of *professional* non-compliance with established guidelines and good practice was noted by Gordis (1979) and emphasised by Ley (1981). Reported rates of professional non-compliance ranged from 12% to 95%, with a median of 80% (Ley 1982). Ley also picked up on the harm caused to patients by the failure of professionals to observe even basic standards of hygiene, especially hand washing (Ley 1997). The extent of nosocomial infections, notably MRSA, is now a topical and increasing problem in modern healthcare systems (Handwashing Liaison Group 1999). However, the irony and double standard involved in professionals expecting patients to comply with medical advice when they themselves routinely do not has been largely overlooked, along with the ethical untenability of such a stance.

A growing body of literature describes the failure of doctors to implement best practice (Schwartz, Soumeris & Ajorn 1989; Weiss & Scott 1997). The proliferation of policy documents and prescribing guidelines, such as National Service Frameworks (www.dh.gov.uk) and National Institute for Clinical Excellence (NICE) reports (www.nice.org.uk), testifies to the concern about standardising clinical procedures and routines. A number of studies have also dealt with the issue of 'irrational' prescribing, particularly the use of antibiotics to treat viral infections. These highlight the importance of a wide range of situational factors as determinants of medical practice. They include the intentional use of the placebo effect, the experience of fatigue or time pressure, and the doctor's desire to protect his relationship with the patient, to avoid conflict in the consultation, or to fulfil what he (often erroneously) perceives to be the patient's expectations (Butler *et al.* 1998; Schwartz, Soumeris & Ajorn 1989; Tomlin, Humphrey & Rogers 1999; Veldhuis, Wigersma & Okkes 1998; Weiss & Scott 1997). This kind of professional non-compliance is directly comparable to patient non-compliance. The situational factors described above are illustrative of the kind of constraints and practical concerns which produce similar kinds of response among both patients and healthcare workers. These are discussed further in Chapter 4.

Unsurprisingly, the professional perspective has tended to focus on the problem of patient non-compliance, and to view this largely as an irrational behaviour resulting from ignorance and/or incompetence. This view derived support from a series of influential studies into patient recall of information carried out by Ley and his associates (Ley 1979a; Ley 1979b; Ley 1982). These found that patients had difficulty remembering much of what doctors told them, and strengthened the widespread professional assumption that patient incompetence was an important cause of failure to take medicines appropriately (Gottleib 2000). This research is the source of the dictum – still frequently reproduced – that as patients can only remember three things they are told in a single consultation there is little point in telling them any more. The assumption that the problem of non-compliance could be solved if patients were sufficiently well informed and consequently able to understand both the instructions accompanying their medicines, as well as the need to take them as prescribed, underpinned the enormous effort that has been poured into interventions to change medicine-taking behaviour through patient education and instruction. Professionals have forgotten the importance which Ley placed on the need for professionals to improve their communication skills and to present information to patients in a clear and accessible manner (Ley 1982). Although non-compliance was usually represented as a result of patient irresponsibility, ignorance or incompetence (Paterson, Russell & Thorne 2001), Ley stressed that it should more appropriately be regarded as due to the failure of professional communication.

In fact, the work of Ley and other researchers in both primary and secondary sectors has consistently found that although patients do forget a substantial amount of what they are told in medical consultations, they still remember a good deal of it: about 60% (Ley 1997). Ley also found that although patients recalled less information in absolute terms, the more extensive and complex the information which they were presented, they still retained the same proportion. Patients who were told more forgot more, but were still better informed than those who received less information. Patients who started off being well informed and knowledgeable were more likely to remember new information presented to them. The findings did not provide a justification for professionals not giving patients good information. However, they did highlight effective communication strategies which doctors could employ in aiding patient recall. For example the sequence of information was important, as patients were more likely to recall what they were told first, and also what they considered to be most important. They also pointed to the importance of contextual factors in determining how well patients remembered and successfully interpreted information. These included the level of anxiety experienced by patients, their previous knowledge and experience of illness, their relationship with the health professional, or whether they were attending for a first or subsequent consultation.

In his more recent analysis (Ley 1997) Ley seems to have taken account of subsequent research and also criticisms that his earlier methodology tended to focus on superficial aspects of patient recall of information rather than the more significant issues of how this was interpreted in relation to their prior knowledge and understanding of the problem (Tuckett et al. 1985). He recognised also that patients' reticence in asking questions reinforces professionals' lack of awareness of their need for information and clarification of what they have been told in medical consultations.

Ley's significant and consistent message has been not that it is pointless to give patients information, but that it is the responsibility of professionals to learn to communicate more effectively. Conceding that organisational and instrumental measures for increasing compliance (such as telephone and written reminders, or improving access and convenience of services) were more effective than didactic ones, Ley emphasises the wider benefits of providing good information to patients, in improving the process of care and increased satisfaction with services (Ley 1982; Ley 1997). In a recent review of the literature Haynes and his colleagues concluded that current methods for improving compliance in chronic conditions require complex and intensive interventions and even then are not particularly effective (McDonald, Garg & Haynes 2002). However, rather than focusing on ways of developing more user-friendly services that patients would find easier to access, much of the more recent compliance research has concentrated instead on ways of reducing intentional non-compliance through effective modification of patient, rather than institutional or professional, behaviour (Heath 2003). From the professional perspective non-compliant patient behaviour appears irrational and intransigent and poses an enduring puzzle.

References

Butler C, Rollnick S, Pill R, Maggs-Rapport F and Stott N (1998) Understanding the culture of prescribing: qualitative study of general practitioners' and patients' perceptions of antibiotics for sore throats. *BMJ.* **317**: 637–42.

Canada AT (1976) The pharmacist and drug compliance. In: DL Sackett and RB Haynes (eds) *Compliance with Therapeutic Regimes.* Johns Hopkins University Press, Baltimore, pp. 129–34.

Carter S, Taylor D and Levenson R (2003) *A Question of Choice – compliance in medicine taking: a preliminary review.* Medicines Partnership, London.

Cochrane AL (1995) Effectiveness and efficiency. In: B Davey, A Gray and C Seale (eds) *Health and Disease: a reader* (2e). Open University Press, Buckingham, pp. 200–207.

Coulter A, Entwistle V and Gilbert D (1998) *Informing Patients: an assessment of the quality of patient information materials.* King's Fund, London.

Coulter A, Entwistle V and Gilbert D (1999) Sharing decisions with patients: is the information good enough? *BMJ.* **318**: 318–22.

Dixon-Woods M (2001) Writing wrongs? An analysis of published discourses about the use of patient information leaflets. *Social Science and Medicine.* **52**(9): 1417–32.

Fitzgerald TD (1976) The influence of the medication on compliance with therapeutic regimens. In: DL Sackett and RB Haynes (eds) *Compliance with Therapeutic Regimes.* Johns Hopkins University Press, Baltimore, pp. 119–28.

Freidson E (1970) *Professional Dominance.* Atherton, New York.

Gibson ES (1979) Compliance and the organization of health services. In: RB Haynes and DL Sackett (eds) *Compliance in Health Care.* Johns Hopkins University Press, Baltimore.

Gordis L (1979) Conceptual and methodologic problems in measuring patent compliance. In: RB Haynes and DL Sackett (eds) *Compliance in Health Care.* Johns Hopkins University Press, Baltimore.

Gottleib H (2000) Medication non-adherence: finding solutions to a costly medical problem. *Drug Benefit Trends.* **12**: 57–62.

Gray R, Wykes T and Gournay K (2002) From compliance to concordance: a review of the literature on interventions to enhance compliance with antipsychotic medication. *Journal of Psychiatric and Mental Health Nursing.* **9**: 277–84.

Handwashing Liaison Group (1999) Handwashing. *BMJ.* **318**: 686.

Haynes B and Haines A (1998) Barriers and bridges to evidence based clinical practice. *BMJ.* **317**(25 July): 273–6.

Haynes R, Devereaux PJ and Guyatt GH (2002) Physicians' and patients' choices in evidence based practice. *BMJ.* **324**: 1350.

Haynes RB (1976a) A critical review of the 'determinants' of patient compliance with therapeutic regimes. In: DL Sackett and RB Haynes (eds) *Compliance with Therapeutic Regimes.* Johns Hopkins University Press, Baltimore, pp. 26–39.

Haynes RB (1976b) Strategies for improving compliance: a methodologic analysis and review. In: DL Sackett and RB Haynes (eds) *Compliance with Therapeutic Regimes.* Johns Hopkins University Press, Baltimore, pp. 69–82.

Haynes RB (1979) Strategies to improve compliance with referrals, appointments and prescribed medical regimes. In: RB Haynes and DL Sackett (eds) *Compliance in Health Care.* Johns Hopkins University Press, Baltimore.

Haynes RB and Sackett DL (1979) *Compliance in Health Care.* Johns Hopkins University Press, Baltimore.

Heath I (2003) A wolf in sheep's clothing: a critical look at the ethics of drug taking. *BMJ.* **327**(11 October): 856–8.

Hogue CC (1979) Nursing and compliance. In: RB Haynes and DL Sackett (eds) *Compliance in Health Care.* Johns Hopkins University Press, Baltimore.

Jonsen AR (1979) Ethical issues in compliance. In: RB Haynes and DL Sackett (eds) *Compliance in Health Care.* Johns Hopkins University Press, Baltimore.

Lerner BH (1997) From careless consumptives to recalcitrant patients: the historical construction of noncompliance. *Social Science and Medicine.* **26**: 577–82.

Ley P (1979a) Improving clinical communication: effects of altering doctor behaviour. In: D Oborne M Gruneberg and J Eiser (eds) *Research in Psychology and Medicine.* Academic Press, London.

Ley P (1979b) The psychology of compliance. In: D Oborne, M Gruneberg and J Eiser (eds) *Research in Psychology and Medicine.* Academic Press, London.

Ley P (1981) Professional non-compliance: a neglected problem. *British Journal of Clinical Psychology.* **20**: 151–4.

Ley P (1982) Satisfaction, compliance and communication. *British Journal of Clinical Psychology.* **21**: 241–54.

Ley P (1997) *Communicating With Patients: improving communication, satisfaction and compliance.* Stanley Thornes (Publishers) Ltd, Cheltenham.

MacPherson R, Jerrom B and Hughes A (1996) A controlled study of education about drug treatment in schizophrenia. *British Journal of Psychiatry.* **168**: 709–17.

McDonald HP, Garg AX and Haynes RB (2002) Interventions to enhance patient adherence to medication prescriptions. *Journal of the American Medical Association.* **288**(22): 2868–79.

McGavock H, Webb HC, Johnston GD and Milligan E (1993) Market penetration of new drugs in one United Kingdom region: implications for general practitioners and administrators. *BMJ.* **307**: 1118–20.

McKenney JM (1979) The clinical pharmacy and compliance. In: RB Haynes and DL Sackett (eds) *Compliance in Health Care.* Johns Hopkins University Press, Baltimore.

Paterson BL, Russell C and Thorne S (2001) Critical analysis of everyday self-care decision making in chronic illness. *Journal of Advanced Nursing.* **35**(3): 335–41.

Sackett DL (1976) Priorities and methods for future research. In: H Sackett and R Haynes (eds) *Compliance in Therapeutic Regimes.* Johns Hopkins University Press, Baltimore, pp. 169–89.

Sackett DL and Haynes R (1976) *Compliance with Therapeutic Regimes*. Johns Hopkins University Press, Baltimore.

Sackett DL, Richardson WS, Rosenberg WMC and Haynes B (1997) *Evidence-Based Medicine: how to practice and teach EBM*. Churchill Livingstone, New York.

Sackett DL, Rosenberg WMC, Muir Gray JA, Haynes R and Richardson WS (1996) Evidence based medicine: what it is and what it isn't. *BMJ*. **312**: 71–2.

Schwartz RK, Soumeris B and Ajorn J (1989) Physician motivations for non-scientific drug prescribing. *Social Science and Medicine*. **28**(6): 577–82.

Tomlin Z, Humphrey C and Rogers S (1999) General practitioners' perceptions of effective health care. *BMJ*. **318**: 1532–5.

Trostle JA (1998) Medical compliance as an ideology. *Social Science and Medicine*. **27**: 1299–1308.

Tuckett D, Boulton M, Olson C and Williams A (1985) *Meetings Between Experts: an approach to sharing ideas in medical consultations*. Tavistock, London.

Veldhuis M, Wigersma L and Okkes I (1998) Deliberate departures from good general practice: a study of motives among Dutch general practitioners. *British Journal of General Practice*. **48**: 1833–6.

Weiss M and Scott D (1997) Whose rationality? A qualitative analysis of general practitioners' prescribing. *Pharmaceutical Journal*. **259**: 339–41.

Chapter Three

Evidence-based medicine

The expectation that patients *should* comply with medical advice, and that they are being uncooperative and/or irrational if they do not, is based on a central assumption that the authority of medical practice derives from the objective and uniform application of scientific principles. This is the basis of medical efficacy and professional expertise. The early work on compliance was sensitive to the need for a highly competent and ethical medical practice in return for public acceptance of professional advice. Patients could only be expected to comply with treatment which was known to be effective, based on accurate diagnosis and to which they had given explicit and properly informed consent (Haynes & Sackett 1979; Sackett & Haynes 1976). However, growing awareness of the extent to which professional practice deviated from these principles stimulated a powerful critique of medicine (see below) and, partly in response to this, the development throughout the 1990s of Evidence-Based Medicine – once again spearheaded by Sackett and Haynes (Cochrane 1999; McAlister *et al.* 2000; Muir Gray 2001; Sackett *et al.* 1996; Sackett *et al.* 1997).

One aspect of the critique of biomedicine focused on the extensive variation in medical practice both between and within countries operating with a similar medical education and culture (Cooper *et al.* 1972; Davis 1994; Davis 1997; Dew 2001; Garratini & Garratini 1993; Muir Gray 2001; Naylor 1995; Payer 1989; Starland 2001; Wahlstrom *et al.* 2002; Wennberg *et al.* 1993). For example, Cooper *et al.* (1972) found that US psychiatrists were more likely to diagnose schizophrenia among their patients than their British counterparts. Payer (1989) gives a very interesting account of the substantial variations in diagnosis and prescribing between doctors in America, France, Germany and the UK. She attributes an important part of these differences in practice between professionals who have been trained within an ostensibly standardised scientific tradition to deeply rooted influences of national culture and history. For example, German doctors make frequent use of a diagnosis 'herzinsuffizienz', relating to a heart complaint which is unrecognised in Britain. They have a much higher prescribing rate for drugs to treat heart disorders compared to their British counterparts, though often use these at a lower dose, but are more conservative in their use of surgery. The incidence of heart disease seems similar in the two populations. Payer attributes these differences in diagnosis and prescribing rates to the deeply engrained associations of the heart with spirituality within German culture.

Other studies have shown that there are substantial variations in practice between different doctors within one country, and even for one individual at different times. The recognition of such variations in medical practice, combined with the realisation that the efficacy of most medical treatments and procedures had never been reliably established (Cochrane 1999; Dew 2001; Elwyn, Edwards & Kinnersley 1999), stimulated the development of Evidence-Based Medicine as a dominant paradigm and continuing legitimator for conventional biomedicine of the present day (Muir Gray 2001) (Box 3.1). It also accounts for the current preoccupation with formulating and implementing national practice guidelines (such as those issued by the National Institute for Clinical Excellence (NICE) in the UK: www.nice.org) as a means of ensuring the standardisation of best practice and its equitable application to all patients.

Box 3.1 Evidence-based medicine

Evidence-based medicine is the conscientious, explicit, and judicious use of current best evidence in making decisions about the care of individual patients. The practice of evidence-based medicine means integrating individual clinical expertise with the best available external clinical evidence from systematic research.

Sackett *et al.* (1996)*

In a landmark publication of 1972, Cochrane drew widespread attention to the extent to which medicine was based on individual clinical experience and traditional practice rather than tested procedures, and proposed the evaluation of practice to be the first priority of the NHS (Cochrane 1999). The randomised control trial (RCT) was advocated as a rigorous and effective method of establishing the effectiveness and efficiency of medical interventions and procedures and a means of determining the 'correct' choice of treatment. The basic principle of the RCT is that randomising subjects between intervention and control groups eliminates the bias inherent in other methods of selection, and provides a secure basis for assessing the therapeutic effects of new and established remedies. Subsequently, the systematic review has been promoted as a rigorous and objective method for evaluating the entire published evidence base for specific interventions. The Cochrane Collaboration has been set up to coordinate a worldwide programme for the conduct and dissemination of reviews (www.update-software.com/publications/cochrane/).

The development of EBM was stimulated by a social and political critique of medical practice originating in the 1960s. Increasing awareness of the harms as well as the benefits of medical treatment was exemplified by high profile tragedies such as the teratogenic effects of thalidomide. The population disease profile shifted as increasing numbers of people lived longer, and with a greater burden of chronic degenerative disease. At the same time, concern arose over the extent to which society was becoming medicalised as professional intervention and control was applied to an increasing range of ordinary problems and experiences of living, such as childbirth or simple unhappiness (Illich 1975; Illich 1977; McNight 1977; Misselbrook & Armstrong 2001; Woivalin *et al.* 2004; Zola 1975; Zola 1977). Freidson (1970) put forward an influential critique of the medical profession which stressed the extent to which medical authority rested on state patronage rather than scientific expertise or therapeutic efficacy. Freidson argued that a

---

* Sackett DL, Rosenberg WMC, Muir Gray JA, Haynes R and Richardson WS (1996) Evidence based medicine: what it is and what it isn't. *BMJ*. **312**: 71–2. Reproduced with permission from the BMJ Publishing Group.

critical attribute of a professional group was that it existed to serve its own interests rather than those of its clients. In return for acting as agents of social control in regulating illness, the medical profession was granted a monopoly of practice, control over recruitment and training, and a considerable degree of autonomy and self-regulation of its members. Increasingly fast information exchange and technological development widened public access to information and began to erode the monopoly over specialist knowledge which had formerly been an important determinant of medical authority. In addition, since the Thatcher government of the early 1980s, there has been growing pressure to achieve increased political accountability and managerial control over medical practice (DHSS 1983; Dopson *et al.* 2003; Misselbrook & Armstrong 2001).

The development of EBM can be interpreted as a response by the medical profession to pressure from a range of different fronts, and an effort to maintain both the credibility and scientific status of clinical practice as well as to retain professional autonomy. The promise of EBM was that doctors would adhere to an internally defined and standardised set of best practices based on compre-hensive and objectively evaluated evidence. Professional autonomy and self-regulation was retained in return for some curtailment of clinical freedom and independence of individual practitioners (Armstrong 2003). EBM has shifted the internal power alignment of the profession in giving prominence to the relatively new and previously marginal discipline of epidemiology (Pope 2003). Some commentators regard the development of EBM as having reinforced the internal divisions within the medical profession, with the medical practice of doctors being increasingly subject to control and regulation by a new medical elite (Armstrong 2003; Pope 2003).

EBM has been highly influential and attractive to policy makers as a means of increasing professional accountability and reducing clinical autonomy, and of promoting visible measures of service evaluation and improvement (Dopson *et al.* 2003). It has stimulated a proliferation of guidelines and practice standards (Pope 2003) which have become an integral part of healthcare. In the UK the establish-ment of the new GP contract from April 2004 links doctors' remuneration to the achievement of specified targets (e.g. statin prescribing) which are supposedly derived from an up-to-date and comprehensive evidence base. However, EBM has also attracted a considerable amount of criticism and resistance – both within the medical profession and outside it. These centre broadly on a critique of the epistemological underpinnings of EBM, the incompatibility of the EBM paradigm with the realities of clinical practice, the opposition between evidence-based practice and clinical autonomy, and the conflict between EBM and another priority area of current health policy: patient-centred medicine and the real-isation of patient choice in healthcare.

EBM developed within a posivitist biomedical paradigm which holds that the natural world is amenable to objective investigation and description. It creates a hierarchy of knowledge within which evidence is ranked in terms of explicit and rigorous rules governing its production and assessment (Cronje & Fullan 2003). The RCT is regarded as the 'gold standard' for testing the effectiveness of medical treatments and procedures. The systematic review of findings has been estab-lished as a means of establishing a definitive evidence base for a particular topic or issue, within which the results of RCTs are deemed to contribute the highest calibre, and most valuable, evidence (Muir Gray 2001; Sackett *et al.* 1997). This simple view of science as capable of producing certain and objective knowledge has been challenged by the constructionist position, which holds that knowledge about the world is not revealed by rigorous investigation but rather is determined by the circumstances and purposes of its production (Berger & Luckmann 1966; Gabbay *et al.* 2003; Harper 1995; Harrison & New 2002). Within this framework EBM can be construed as an attempt to impose stability and discipline on the uncertainty and variability of medical practice (Dew 2001; Pope 2003).

While the proposition that medicine should be based on a sound evidence base seems uncontestable, the constructionist critique of EBM questions the status of the 'evidence' as an artefact rather than 'reality'. It is argued that research interests and activity are driven by historical contingencies as well as powerful commercial interests which direct the focus of investigation away from the complex processes of healthcare delivery that are of greatest import-ance to patients. Instead, most research is dictated by the needs of the pharmaceutical companies to test new pharmaceutical products, and it is in this area that most RCTs are carried out (Harrison & New 2002). Concerns have been raised about the distortion of evidence resulting from publication bias prompted by the tendency to conceal or withhold negative findings (Rogers 2002).

RCTs are undertaken under tightly defined conditions, and with carefully selected participants (e.g. not too young, not too old, not too ill) who may bear little relation to the kind of complex case for whom new treatments or interventions will be prescribed in the context of normal medical practice (Black 1996; Dieppe *et al.* 2004; Naylor 1995; Pope 2003; Starland 2001; Stricker & Psaty 2004). Decisions about criteria of inclusion, exclusion and outcome assessment are arbitrary, but nevertheless determine the evidence produced by the review. In addition, RCTs deal with data that can be easily measured and quantified, which exclude large areas of healthcare relating to complex processes of service delivery and evaluation (Ford, Schofield & Hope 2002; Rogers 2002). Cochrane himself recognised that there are many areas of medical practice, such as psychiatry, where RCTs cannot be applied (Cochrane 1999; Faulkener & Thomas 2002). However, the focus on EBM has supported the routing of research funds and effort in psychiatry to the testing of psychiatric drugs, rather than the evaluation of alternative forms of treatment, such as psychological and talking therapies, which may not only be effective options, but also more highly valued by patients (Rogers 2002).

Systematic reviews tend to be carried out in areas where there is already a considerable amount of evidence to examine, and so focus attention on existing knowledge rather than the exploration of what is not known. Moreover, the weighting of evidence in terms of 'quality' accorded to different methodologies effectively leads to the exclusion of much available research, including the findings of qualitative studies (Booth 2001; Dixon-Woods & Fitzpatrick 2001). In the past, these have been regarded as near the bottom of the knowledge hierarchy. The value of qualitative findings is now increasingly recognised, and efforts are being made to develop systems for incorporating them within system-atic reviews (Dixon-Woods *et al.* 2004; Dixon-Woods & Fitzpatrick 2001; Thomas *et al.* 2004). However, given the radically different epistemological and metho-dological starting points of qualitative and positivistic research, it is not yet clear how this can be achieved.

Recognition of the insights which can be generated by qualitative studies has served to highlight that there are different *kinds* of evidence which need to be taken into account, including those, such as patients' accounts and interpretations of illness experience, which cannot be measured (Cronje & Fullan 2003; Harper 1995; Sullivan & MacNaughton 1996). These call for different criteria of appraisal and analysis, but can be at least as rigorous and credible as those of systematic reviews. Cronje and Fullan (2003) differentiate 'practical' ways of knowing based on the expert judgement and consensus from 'scientific' knowing based on the application of rules. A constructionist critique of EBM proposes that a rules-based system of appraisal merely masks the judgements and decisions which underpin the system. Qualitative analysis, in contrast, endeavours to expose subjectivity and make such underlying assumptions explicit.

The high policy and academic profile of EBM has not been matched by a corresponding change in medical culture and professional practice. Although deriving much of its authority from an ostensible basis in scientific evidence and enquiry, biomedicine has always been applied pragmatically. The conflict between the restrictive and standardising tendencies of EBM and the deeply entrenched traditions of clinical judgement and practitioner autonomy account for a good deal of the resistance which has arisen within professional medicine, and the failure of EBM to be widely applied in practice (Armstrong 2003; Cronje & Fullan 2003; Dew 2001; Feinstein 1976; Feinstein 1994; Gabbay *et al.* 2003; Naylor 1995; Pope 2003; Schwartz, Soumeris & Ajorn 1989).

In addition to the professional resistance to the infringement of clinical autonomy, it is evident that the gulf between evidence and practice derives substantially from the contingencies and complexities of the real world. Statistical generalisations based on aggregate data often cannot be satisfactorily applied to the particularities of individual cases (Pope 2003; Starland 2001). RCTs might establish standards of evidence, but medical decisions involve judgements which are underpinned by values and the convictions of experience (Dew 2001; Feinstein 1976; Feinstein 1994; Gabbay, le May, Jefferson, Webb, Lovelock, Powell & Lathlean 2003; Pope 2003). Studies of medical practice reveal the nature and influence of situational constraints on consultation outcomes. Factors such as shortage of time, complex co-morbidity, scarcity of resources and the doctor's desire to avoid conflict and protect his relationship with patients can all get in the way of evidence-based medicine. Thus different rationalities of practice apply in different contexts. Realising the best outcome in particular circumstances may involve deviating from objectively defined 'best' practice (Rees Jones *et al.* 2004; Schwartz, Soumeris & Ajorn 1989; Tomlin, Humphrey & Rogers 1999; Veldhuis, Wigersma & Okkes 1998).

The prescriptive guidelines derived from evidence-based practice also conflict with the priority to develop patient-centred medicine (PCM) which takes account of individual choice and preferences (Bensing 2000; Ford, Schofield & Hope 2002; Lewis, Robinson & Wilkinson 2003; Rogers 2002). Armstrong (2003) suggests that the rhetoric of patient-centred medicine functions as a form of professional resistance to evidence-based medicine. In recent publications Sackett and other proponents of EBM have acknowledged, perhaps rather belatedly, that clinical judgement and patient preferences have always been essential components of good care (Haynes, Devereaux & Guyatt 2002; Sackett *et al.* 1996). EBM serves merely to inform decisions and ensure that these are based on the most reliable available knowledge. However, it is difficult to see how these opposing paradigms may be combined. In focusing on defined disease categories and specific interventions EBM overlooks the *process* of healthcare and its importance to patients' experience and evaluation of treatment. Moreover, particularly in general practice, professionals are often faced with problems that are vague and indeterminate and elude the application of discrete labels and situations in which the best or most appropriate treatment is unclear (Naylor 1995). In conceding this point, EBM loses much of its force; in resisting, it loses much of its relevance.

The accelerated pace of technological innovation has produced a range of therapeutic options, but often the outcomes of these are uncertain or imperfectly understood. Paradoxically, evidence-based medicine often uncovers the marginal gains to be made between different treatments, while exposing the fine balance between benefits and risk (Barry *et al.* 1988; Wennberg *et al.* 1993). The divisions and uncertainties within medicine, the contested nature of findings and research are widely circulated through the media. In such a context, the 'expert' role of the professional becomes increasingly hard to sustain and legitimise. Clinical variation and medical uncertainty reveal the weakness of the scientific basis of much medical practice, and expose the extent to which medical decisions rest on the application of practitioner values and judgements. Where this is the case, it is difficult to justify the exclusion of patients from participation in choices and decisions about treatment and illness management that significantly affect them. There is no good reason for continuing to privilege professional over lay judgement.

The 'best' decision in a given situation is often contextually and culturally determined, and may rest – crucially – on the goals and values of the patient. In fact, patients are accustomed to making choices about treatment – and these are manifest in the very high rates of 'non-compliance' with medical advice. A central assumption of patient-centred medicine and concordance is that the development of a better understanding between patients and professionals, and in particular, a greater awareness by professionals firstly that patients *have* a perspective on illness management, and secondly of what this is, will enable them to improve the quality of healthcare by assisting patients to make better and more informed choices about treatment. Such an understanding will also engender a satisfactory explanation of why patients do not comply with treatment.

References

Armstrong D (2003) Clinical autonomy, individual and collective: the problem of changing doctors' behaviour. *Social Science and Medicine.* **55**(10): 1771–7.

Barry MJ, Mulley AG, Fowler FJ and Wennberg JW (1988) Watchful waiting vs immediate transurethral resection for symptomatic prostatism. *Journal of the American Medical Association.* **259**: 3010–17.

Bensing J (2000) Bridging the gap. The separate worlds of evidence-based medicine and patient-centred medicine. *Patient Education and Counselling.* **39**: 17–25.

Berger PL and Luckmann T (1966) *The Social Construction of Reality.* Penguin, Harmondsworth.

Black N (1996) Why we need observational studies to evaluate the effectiveness of health care. *BMJ.* **312**(11): 1215–18.

Booth A (2001) *Cochrane or Cock-eyed? How Should We Conduct Systematic Reviews of Qualitative Research?* Paper presented at the Qualitative Evidence-based Practice Conference, Taking a Critical Stance, Coventry University, 14–16 May. 25-8-2004.

Cochrane AL (1999) *Effectiveness and Efficiency: random reflections on health services*. The Royal Society of Medicine Press, London.

Cooper J, Kendall RE, Gurland BJ, Sharpe L, Copeland JRM and Simon R (1972) *Psychiatric Diagnosis in New York and London*. Oxford University Press, London.

Cronje R and Fullan A (2003) Evidence-based medicine: toward a new definition of 'rational' medicine. *Health*. **7**(3): 353–69.

Davis P (1994) Accounting for variation in drug therapy. In: G Harding, S Nettleton and K Taylor (eds) *Social Pharmacy, Innovation and Development*. The Pharmaceutical Press, London, pp. 130–43.

Davis P (1997) *Managing Medicines*. Open University Press, Buckingham.

Dew K (2001) Models of practice and models of science in medicine. *Health*. **5**(1): 93–111.

DHSS (1983) *NHS Management Inquiry* (The Griffiths Management Report). DHSS, London.

Dieppe P, Bartlett C, Davey P, Doyal L and Ebrahim S (2004) Balancing benefits and harms: the example of non-steroidal anti-inflammatory drugs. BMJ. **329**(3 July): 31–4.

Dixon-Woods M, Agarwal S, Young B, Jones D and Sutton AJ (2004) *Integrative Approaches to Qualitative and Quantitative Evidence*. Health Development Agency, London.

Dixon-Woods M and Fitzpatrick R (2001) Qualitative research in systematic reviews. *BMJ*. **323**(6 October): 765.

Dopson S, Locock L, Gabbay J, Ferlie E and Fitzgerald L (2003) Evidence-based medicine and the implementation gap. *Health*. **7**(3): 311–30.

Elwyn G, Edwards A and Kinnersley P (1999) Shared decision-making in primary care: the neglected second half of the consultation. *British Journal of General Practice*. **49**: 477–82.

Faulkener A and Thomas P (2002) User-led research and evidence-based medicine. *British Journal of Psychiatry*. **180**: 1–3.

Feinstein AR (1976) 'Compliance bias' and the interpretation of therapeutic trials. In: DL Sackett and RB Haynes (eds) *Compliance with Therapeutic Regimes*. Johns Hopkins University Press, Baltimore, pp. 152–66.

Feinstein AR (1994) Clinical judgement revisited: the distraction of quantitative models. *Annals of Internal Medicine*. **120**: 799–805.

Ford S, Schofield T and Hope T (2002) Barriers to the evidence-based patient choice (EBPC) consultation. *Patient Education and Counselling*. **47**: 179–85.

Freidson E (1970) *Professional Dominance*. Atherton, New York.

Gabbay J, le May A, Jefferson H, Webb D, Lovelock R, Powell J and Lathlean J (2003) A case study of knowledge management in multi-agency consumer-informed 'communities of practice': implications for evidence-based policy development in health and social services. *Health*. **7**(3): 283–310.

Garratini S and Garratini L (1993) Pharmaceutical prescriptions in four European countries. *Lancet*. **342**: 1191–2.

Harper D (1995) Discourse analysis and 'mental health'. *Journal of Mental Health*. **4**(4): 347–8.

Harrison A and New B (2002) *Public Interest, Private Decisions: health-related research in the UK*. King's Fund, London.

Haynes R, Devereaux PJ and Guyatt GH (2002) Physicians' and patients' choices in evidence based practice. *BMJ*. **324**: 1350.

Haynes RB and Sackett DL (1979) *Compliance in Health Care*. Johns Hopkins University Press, Baltimore.

Illich I (1975) *Medical Nemesis*. Caldar and Boyars, London.

Illich I (1977) Disabling professions. In: I Illich *et al.* (eds) *Disabling Professions*. Marion Boyars Publishers, London, pp. 11–39.

Lewis DK, Robinson J and Wilkinson E (2003) Factors involved in deciding to start preventive treatment: qualitative study of clinicians' and lay people's attitudes. *BMJ*. **327**(11 October): 841.

McAlister FA, Straus SE, Guyatt GH and Haynes RB (2000) Users' Guides to the Medical Literature XX integrating research evidence with the care of the individual patient. *Journal of the American Medical Association.* **283**(21): 2829–36.

McNight J (1977) Professionalized service and disabling help. In: I Illich *et al.* (eds) *Disabling Professions.* Marion Boyars Publishers, London, pp. 69–92.

Misselbrook D and Armstrong D (2001) Patients' responses to risk information about the benefits of treating hypertension. *British Journal of General Practice.* **51**: 276–9.

Muir Gray JA (2001) Evidence-based medicine for professionals. In: A Edwards and G Elwyn (eds) *Evidence-Based Patient Choice, Inevitable or Impossible?* Oxford University Press, Oxford, pp. 19–33.

Naylor DC (1995) Grey zones of clinical practice: some limits to evidence-based medicine. *Lancet.* **345**(8953): 840–3.

Payer L (1989) *Medicine and Culture: notions of health and sickness in Britain, the US, France and Germany.* Victor Gollanz Ltd, London.

Pope C (2003) Resisting evidence: the study of evidence-based medicine as a contemporary social movement. *Health.* **7**(3): 267–82.

Rees Jones I, Berney L, Kelly M, Doyal L, Griffiths C, Feder G, Hillier S, Rowlands G and Curtis S (2004) Is patient involvement possible when decisions involve scarce resources? A qualitative study of decision-making in primary care. *Social Science and Medicine.* **59**: 93-102.

Rogers WA (2002) Evidence-based medicine in practice: limiting or facilitating patient choice? *Health Expectations.* **5**: 95–103.

Sackett DL and Haynes R (1976) *Compliance with Therapeutic Regimes.* Johns Hopkins University Press, Baltimore.

Sackett DL, Richardson WS, Rosenberg WMC and Haynes B (1997) *Evidence-Based Medicine: how to practice and teach EBM.* Churchill Livingstone, New York.

Sackett DL, Rosenberg WMC, Muir Gray JA, Haynes R and Richardson WS (1996) Evidence based medicine: what it is and what it isn't. *BMJ.* **312**: 71–2.

Schwartz RK, Soumeris B and Ajorn J (1989) Physician motivations for non-scientific drug prescribing. *Social Science and Medicine.* **28**(6): 577–82.

Starland B (2001) New paradigms for quality in primary care. *British Journal of General Practice.* **51**: 303–9.

Stricker BH and Psaty BM (2004) Detection, verification, and quantification of adverse drug reactions. *BMJ.* **329**(3 July): 44–7.

Sullivan FM and MacNaughton RJ (1996) Evidence in consultations: interpreted and individualised. *Lancet.* **348**(9032): 941–4.

Thomas J, Harden A, Oakley A, Oliver S, Sutcliffe K, Rees R, Brunton G and Kavanagh J (2004) Integrating qualitative research with trials in systematic reviews. *BMJ.* **328**(24 April): 1010–12.

Tomlin Z, Humphrey C and Rogers S (1999) General practitioners' perceptions of effective health care. *BMJ.* **318**: 1532–5.

Veldhuis M, Wigersma L and Okkes I (1998) Deliberate departures from good general practice: a study of motives among Dutch general practitioners. *British Journal of General Practice.* **48**: 1833–6.

Wahlstrom R, Hummers-Pradier E, Stalsby Lundborg C, Muskova M, Lagerlov P, Denig P, Oke T, Chaput de Saintonage DM and the Drug Education Project group (2002) Variations in asthma treatment in five European countries – judgement analysis of case simulations. *Family Practice.* **19**(5): 452–60.

Wennberg JE, Barry MJ, Fowler FJ and Mulley A (1993) Outcomes research, PORTs and health care reform. *Annals New York Academy of Sciences.* **703**: 52–62.

Woivalin T, Krantz G, Mantyranta T and Ringsberg KC (2004) Medically unexplained symptoms: perceptions of physicians in primary health care. *Family Practice.* **21**(2): 199–203.

Zola IK (1975) Medicine as an institution of social control. In: C Cox and A Mead (eds) *A Sociology of Medical Practice*. Collier-MacMillan, London, pp. 170–246.

Zola IK (1977) Healthism and disabling medicalization. In: I Illich *et al.* (eds) *Disabling Professions*. Marion Boyars Publishers, London, pp. 41–68.

Chapter Four

The lay perspective

Introduction

The professional construction of compliance and the development of EBM developed from within the culture of mainstream biomedical research and practice. Running in parallel to this from the 1970s onwards, a growing body of sociological work started to reveal the existence and complexity of lay concepts of health underlying illness behaviour (Backett 1992; Blaxter 1982; Cornwell 1985; Crawford 1984; Herzlich 1973; Pill & Stott 1982; Pollock 1993). The development of 'grounded theory' was a powerful tool of qualitative research which involved an intensive scrutiny of respondents' verbatim accounts. The aim was to develop concepts inductively, and build theory from 'the ground up' (Strauss & Corbin 1998). This contrasted with the hypothetico-deductive method ('top down' approach) characteristic of conventional scientific research, which proceeded through the systematic formulation and testing of predetermined hypotheses. Sociological interest at this time extended from the analysis of medical systems and formal healthcare to an investigation of the experience of health and illness in everyday life, and the illness behaviour of individual patients (Anderson & Bury 1988; Stimson & Webb 1975; Wadsworth & Robinson 1976). One of the striking findings was not only the high prevalence of symptoms among the population at any time, but also how infrequently these prompted visits to the doctor (Dunnell & Cartwright 1972; Hannay 1979; Wadsworth, Butterfield & Blaney 1971). Dunnell and Cartwright (1972) found that 91% of adult respondents had experienced symptoms during the preceding fortnight and each reported an average of 3.9 symptoms. Wadsworth, Butterfield & Blaney (1971) found that 95% of 2153 respondents reported health complaints but less than a third of those reporting at least one painful or distressing symptom had contacted their doctor during this time. Hannay (1979) found not only that most people did not consult about most of their symptoms (especially mental problems) but that nearly a quarter of people reporting symptoms they considered to be severe or serious did not seek medical advice. He called this phenomenon 'the symptom iceberg'.

It became apparent that most illnesses – including quite serious conditions – were handled much of the time within the lay sector, and did not reach the attention of health professionals. Wadsworth, Butterfield & Blaney (1971) found that most (68%) illnesses had been first diagnosed by the patient rather than the doctor. Medicine taking was common, with over the counter (OTC) products being taken twice as often as prescribed ones. Even so, Dunnell and Cartwright found that no treatment was accessed for almost half (47%) of all symptoms. People were seen to be active managers of their health, making their own judgements about how to treat illness, and when it was necessary to consult a doctor for advice. They did not cease to monitor and evaluate their condition, including any treatment that had been prescribed, after they left the consulting room (Stimson & Webb 1975; West 1976). This research shed a new light on why patients did not take their medicines as their doctors advised and exposed the extent to which lay and professional goals and values could differ from each other.

Ideas of health and illness

The importance of health to personal identity, and people's sense of personal competence and autonomy, became apparent (Charmaz 1983; Cornwell 1985; Good 1994; Herzlich 1973; Pollock 1993; Williams 1983). Health was revealed as a social (rather than medical) construct loaded with moral value and personal significance. It was commonly regarded both as a means to continuing social and economic functioning, rather than as an end in itself, and as the visible expression of personal competence and integrity (Blaxter 1993; Williams 1993). People occupied the role of patient intermittently and transiently and, except in extreme cases, this did not constitute a major determinant of their social status or personal identity. Where the requirements of healthy living conflicted with other goals and obligations, as was frequently the case, it was often the latter that were prioritised (Backett 1992). The commitment to health as a value, combined with a normatively functional definition of health (capacity to carry out normal roles and responsibilities) enabled people to maintain that their health was *good*, despite the fact that they suffered from severe or incapacitating illness (Dunnell & Cartwright 1972; Kagawa-Singer 1993; Pollock 1993; Wadsworth, Butterfield & Blaney 1971). For example, Pollock (1993) found that despite being severely physically disabled by MS, respondents could still categorise their health as good, because of the separation they effected between their core self and the illness. As long as the mind retained its integrity, the essential person remained unscathed, and could even become stronger in response to the challenge of illness and adversity. Similarly, Kagawa-Singer (1993) found that cancer patients also considered themselves to have good health, because this was defined in terms of functional capacity and social involvement, rather than absence of disease.

Kagawa-Singer's comparison of Anglo-Americans and Japanese-Americans revealed some differences in responses to cancer, though both groups expressed a concept of health based on a sense of self-integrity manifest through social engagement rather than bodily disorder. For example, Anglo-Americans tended to resent the intrusion of cancer into their lives, which they viewed as originating in arbitrary factors external to themselves. The Japanese-Americans, in contrast, tended to locate the source of the illness in intrinsic factors relating to their earlier experiences and lifestyle choices. This is attributed to differences in the characteristic orientations of each cultural group in responding to misfortune. The Japanese concept of karma entails acceptance of personal responsibility for adversity, and stoical endurance. In contrast, the Anglo-American response was typically one of externalising the illness as an adversary. Anglo-American respondents dug deep into their inner resources of will power and determination to resist or 'fight' their illness. Japanese-Americans tended to adopt a more passive strategy of avoidance and repression of their anxieties and emotions in preserving a façade of normality. Kagawa-Singer regards this kind of coping strategy as a positive use of denial to enable the continuation of hope and the illusion of normality in the face of serious illness.

Illness narratives

Kagawa-Singer's study illustrates the range of different coping strategies adopted by the same person at different points in time, and also the influence of culture in shaping illness responses and providing a repertoire of options for individuals to draw on in accounting for misfortune. In a classic anthropological monograph describing illness beliefs among the Azande in Africa, Evans-Pritchard highlighted the significance which people place on accounting for 'the particularity of misfortune' (Evans-Pritchard 1937). Scientific descriptions of disease may offer an understanding of cause and process, but they do nothing to explain the contingencies of affliction: why me? why now? Lay perspectives do not lack awareness of the natural processes and determinants of disease. However, they are more urgently focused on the need to invest meaning, and consequently also a degree of coherence and sense of control, over arbitrary and chaotic events and experiences which threaten not only the body, but also the self.

A considerable body of research has focused on the role of the patient's story, or narrative, and its importance as a means of making sense of illness (Bury 2001; Elwyn & Gwyn 1999; Good 1994; Hyden 1997; Kangas 2001; Kleinman 1988; Radley 1993; Williams 1984; Williams 1993). Blaxter (1982, 1983, 1993) examined accounts of health and illness among three generations of working class women in North West Scotland. Her respondents made sense of their current health in terms of previous illness episodes and life experiences. The experience of health and illness was integrated within a connected biography, in which one health condition was often seen to result, or run on from, an earlier illness or experience. The demands of childbearing were held to have a particularly strong bearing on susceptibility to ill health in later life. Williams (1993) described a similar process of 'narrative reconstruction' among a group of elderly arthritis sufferers. The 'genesis' of their illness was embedded in the trajectory of their life course, which could be reviewed and reinterpreted to explain, and confer meaning, on an otherwise arbitrary and inexplicable event. A central task of patient narratives was to express or confirm the continuing integrity and moral virtue of the individual as this was revealed in his *response* to illness, which, unlike its occurrence, was to a considerable extent volitional.

Morris observes that 'illness threatens to undo our sense of who we are' (1998: 22).* Williams (1984) views narrative reconstruction as a means of responding to this 'biographical disruption' (Bury 1982) of illness and repairing the breaches it poses to personal identity and ontological security. Good (1994) comments on the plasticity of the narrative form, and also its avoidance of ending or closure. This enables individual stories to respond flexibly to new knowledge and events, and also to incorporate and selectively attend to disparate strands of cause and consequence. Launer (2002) similarly characterises the narrative as a 'situated discourse': formed and varied in response to the context and circumstances of its production, whether this is a research interview, medical consultation, or social conversation.

Kleinman (1988) picks up on the communicative function of patient narrative, as a personal expression of distress and a bridge to shared experience and

* From DB Morris *Illness and Culture in the Postmodern Age.* © 1998 The Regents of the University of California.

empathetic witnessing of suffering (Frank 1995; Hyden & Peolsson 2002). In these accounts, lay narratives also feature as a means of articulating *resistance* to impersonal biomedical accounts of disease, in which the patient's experience and articulation of illness is largely bypassed and ignored. We will look again at the consequences of this opposition between lay and professional narratives in Chapter 9. However, the preceding discussion has underlined the distance between patient concerns about the experience of *illness* and the biomedical focus on treating *disease*. It also points to substantial differences between patients and professionals in the values, objectives and concerns that frame the ways in which medicines are prescribed and used.

Medicines

Research into how patients with severe and chronic illness cope with their symptoms reveals the complexity of management strategies they employ, and the effort that is put into 'normalising' the condition. A precariously negotiated balance has to be struck between incapacity and autonomy. The effort to stay at work, to carry out normal domestic roles and responsibilities and engage in social activities – in short, to continue to be the same person as before the illness – is paramount (Anderson & Bury 1988; Arluke 1980; Charmaz 1983; Conrad 1997; Donovan & Blake 1992; Pollock 1993; Wright 2000). Ill health is a highly disvalued social state. Medicines may be regarded as a means of restoring or maintaining health, or alternatively as an unwelcome signifier of impairment: sometimes both (Conrad 1985). Medicines frequently produce unwelcome side effects. Their use may be hard to conceal or felt to be stigmatising. In such circumstances, the patient's decision not to 'comply' with medical advice can be seen as a means of realising more important goals, rather than a failure to act rationally. The key issue here is that patient and professional definitions of 'best interest' may differ, in accordance with the different values and goals to be pursued. Thus, what appears to be irrational behaviour in medical terms can be regarded as entirely rational – 'reasoned decision-making' from within the patient's perspective (Arluke 1980; Donovan & Blake 1992).

The demographic disease profile in industrialised countries has changed from a preponderance of acute to chronic degenerative disorders. As a result, it is common for people to face the prospect of living a substantial part of their lives with at least one long-term illness, for which they are likely to be prescribed at least one medicine. The extent of medicine taking is enormous: the Medicines Partnership website (www.medicines-partnership.org) states that 70% of the UK population is taking medicines at any one time and similarly high figures have been proposed by others (Asscher, Parr & Whitmarsh 1995; Coleman 2003; Davis 1997). Payer's analysis suggests that Britain has a more restrained and conservative approach to prescribing than other comparable European countries or the US (Davis 1997; Payer 1989). Even so, driven by aggressive commercial and professional interests, medicines have become an enormously powerful personal and social technology, assuming great symbolic as well as therapeutic significance (Chetley 1990; Cohen *et al.* 2001; de Joncheere *et al.* 2003; Dowell & Hudson 1997; Morgan 1996; Pellegrino 1976; Vuckovic & Nichter 1997). Seventy per cent of GP consultations are reported to end with a prescription, with the average person receiving seven to eight scripts a year (Davis 1997).

The benefits of medicines can be great, and so can their harms (Asscher, Parr & Whitmarsh 1995; Briceland 2000; Cohen *et al.* 2001; Institute of Medicine 2000; Sandars & Esmail 2003; Starland 2001). A recent review by Pirmohamed *et al.* (2004) found that 6.5% of UK hospital admissions were related to adverse drug reactions (ADR), with the ADR leading directly to admission in 80% of cases. This figure corresponds closely to the findings of earlier studies (Asscher, Parr & Whitmarsh 1995; Institute of Medicine 2000). Older people are particularly vulnerable to suffering harm from their medicines. Heath (Heath 2003) cites evidence from an American study which estimates that up to 28% of hospital admissions for elderly patients in the US are related to adverse drug reactions: ADRs appear to cause a great deal more harm than patient non-compliance, as well as being themselves an important reason for patients not to take their medicines as prescribed.

These figures relate only to reported events involving hospital admissions. The scale of unrecognised and unreported errors and ADRs in the community is likely to be very substantially larger. Sandars and Esmail (2003) concluded that pre-scribing and prescription errors have been identified in up to 11% of all UK prescriptions, mainly relating to dose. Particularly within the field of mental health, user surveys have revealed the frequency and extent to which the side effects of drugs used to treat psychiatric disorders substantially impair patients' quality of life (Campbell, Cobb & Darton 1998; Cobb, Darton & Kiran 2001; Corry, Hogman & Sandamas 2002; Day, Kinderman & Benthall 1998; Petit-Zeman, Sandamas & Hogman 2001; Rogers & Pilgrim 1993). Cohen *et al.* (2001) comment on a paradox of modern pharmaceuticals: accepted as a triumph and technolo-gical wonder whilst actually constituting a major cause of morbidity and mortality, and ranking as the fourth to sixth leading cause of death in US hospitals (see also Misselbrook 2001). Given the scale of inappropriate or harmful prescribing, the frequency of adverse effects and the inability to anticipate either the optimum dose or physiological response for any given individual, it may be that non-compliance and personal experimentation is an effective strategy in helping to reduce the extent of overmedication and experience of adverse drug reactions (Donovan 1995; Heath 2003).

Given the real risk and often doubtful or uncertain efficacy, it is clear that patients have good grounds for caution in accepting and using medicines. The experience of side effects, and concerns about future harm resulting from long-term use are important reasons why patients want to limit their consumption. However, side effects may be tolerated, even when severe, if the benefits are considered to outweigh the disadvantages (Hogman & Sandamas 2000; Rogers *et al.* 1998). Pragmatic concerns relating to the effort to maintain a normal life and protect important goals and valued activities are also an important determinant of medicine-taking behaviour. In his study of patients' use of drugs to control epilepsy, Conrad (1985) found that respondents were less likely to tolerate side effects which jeopardised their capacity to carry on their normal roles and social activities and obligations than the experience of physical discomfort.

A number of studies describe the situational manipulation of medicine taking so that side and/or therapeutic effects would fit in with life events and routines (Morgan 1996). Symptoms may only need to be controlled, or side effects avoided, in certain contexts or situations. For example, respondents in Rogers *et al.*'s study (1998) reported taking neuroleptic medication when they felt the need to control their symptoms and appear 'normal' to others. Another response was to leave off taking tablets before embarking on a planned episode of social drinking. In this context it is hard to argue that adherence to medication is more important than continued social participation. Conrad (1997) describes the adjustment made by one respondent (a student) who reported taking more of his epilepsy treatment immediately before sitting an exam, to ensure that he was clear headed and secure from seizures at this time. Another example is provided where a respondent only took antihistamines to control the symptoms of hay fever while at work, where she felt the disruption these would otherwise cause was unacceptable (Britten 1994).

These studies indicate that patients' medicine taking is often oriented to the *control* or *management* of symptoms, rather than their elimination. In particular, it appears that being free of symptoms may be less important than maintaining at least the appearance of normality. Thus, if people perceive the side effects or visibility of their medicine taking to impair their ability to engage in valued relationships and activities, they are likely to alter their prescribed regimen (Conrad 1985; Conrad 1997; Pound *et al.* 2005; Rogers *et al.* 1998). The converse, of course, is also true.

Sometimes difficult equations have to be made between the costs and benefits of treatment. For example, Rogers *et al.* (1998) describe the dilemma for patients prescribed neuroleptics to control the symptoms of schizophrenia. The trade-off to be made here is the important gain of staying out of hospital, against the experience of unpleasant and debilitating side effects together with the anticipation of a substantially reduced lifespan. In this context the extent to which patients value being able to retain their social and economic involvement and responsibilities can be an important determinant of adherence.

In managing their illness, patients sometimes want to test out the extent of their recovery, the efficacy of their medicines, and possibly also the accuracy of their doctors, by seeing what happens when they stop the treatment. Several studies have reported that patients stop treatment once they are feeling better, or because they have been continuing on it for some time, or because they have concerns that prolonged use of specific drugs will result in loss of therapeutic efficacy. They fear that their bodies will become 'resistant' and wish to retain a degree of therapeutic credit saved against future need (Arluke 1980; Donovan & Blake 1992; Dunnell & Cartwright 1972; Fallsberg 1991). These forms of experimentation and treatment self-regulation constitute a rational strategy, as patients continually reappraise the efficacy of their treatments, and the necessity of continuing to take their medicines (Arluke 1980; Conrad 1985; Donovan 1995; Dowell & Hudson 1997; Fallsberg 1991; Pound *et al.* 2005; Stevenson *et al.* 2000).

Neither concern about side effects nor the pragmatic strategies of illness management discussed above are sufficient to explain the widespread lay aversion to medicine taking which is widely documented throughout the literature (Adams, Pill & Jones 1997; Arluke 1980; Benson & Britten 2002; Britten 1994; Britten *et al.* 2004; Conrad 1985; Donovan & Blake 1992; Dowell & Hudson 1997; Fallsberg 1991; Hunter & Britten 1997; Lewis, Robinson & Wilkinson 2003; Lisper *et al.* 1997; Pound *et al.* 2005; Rogers *et al.* 1998; Stevenson *et al.* 2000; Townsend, Hunt & Wyke 2003). This is derived from deeply ingrained cultural norms defining personal competence and autonomy and appropriate responses to illness. Part of the ambivalence towards medicines stems from their dual role in signifying illness as well as legitimating it (Arluke 1980; Benson & Britten 2002; Britten 1994; Cornwell 1985; Donovan & Blake 1992; Fallsberg 1991; Townsend, Hunt & Wyke 2003). Medicines can help to sustain normality but also signify impairment and vulnerability. In Morgan's study (Morgan 1996), for example, respondents rejected the status of illness signified by the diagnosis of hypertension, but were uneasy about the ambiguous health status they now occupied as a result of having to take long-term medication.

The experience of illness constitutes a serious challenge to the experience of the self as an integrated and continuing entity (Charmaz 1983). One of the important issues for many patients is the degree to which they can maintain control over their illness symptoms, and also, by extension, themselves. Medicines promise personal control over illness and freedom from pain and discomfort. They may constitute a convenient and effective coping mechanism in enabling people to overcome potentially disabling discomfort and distress, and be valued accordingly. For many, however, the fact that medicines are required to realise such freedom signifies that medicine taking is itself an indication of dependency. Patients will often tolerate considerable pain and discomfort in preference for remaining actively in charge of their health. Donovan (1995) found that four fifths of her respondents said they would do anything rather than take drugs for their arthritis. Non-adherence to medicines can thus be an adaptive coping strategy where it enhances the individual's sense of autonomy and ability not to let either medicines or illness assume undue control over their lives (Arluke 1980; Conrad 1997; Donovan & Blake 1992; Fallsberg 1991; Stevenson, Wallance, Rivers & Gerrett 2000; Townsend, Hunt & Wyke 2003). Effectively, patients may be operating with a different concept and criteria of efficacy from their doctors. Their intentional and reasoned experiments with medicine taking are undertaken as part of an attempt to realise their individual perceptions of the best available quality of life.

Medicines can impact in complex ways on patients' experience of identity and sense of wellbeing. They are commonly regarded as a 'necessary evil' (Stevenson, Wallance, Rivers & Gerrett 2000; Townsend, Hunt & Wyke 2003). People may value the benefits of medicines in enabling the restoration or maintenance of their normal lives and selves, but resent their ongoing need and incapacity to do without. The iatrogenic consequences of medicine taking in extending beyond purely physiological damage to undermine self-efficacy have long been recognised (Illich 1975; Zola 1975; Zola 1977). Misselbrook (2001) discusses the negative impact of modern medicine in damaging patients' perceptions of their health and undermining their sense of wellbeing. For example, once the label of 'hypertensive' has been attached to them, people are likely to feel and behave as unhealthy, with a decline in motivation and increased work absenteeism (Blumhagen 1980; Davis 1997; Haynes 1979). This is so, even when the condition targeted for detection and treatment is merely a risk factor, rather than overt disease. Similarly, Sachs (1995) describes the problematic experience of men in whom raised cholesterol levels had been detected as they struggled to 'visualise the invisible' and come to terms with the existence of 'unfelt pathology'. Their bodily experience of being well and vigorous is revealed as untrustworthy, and overridden by the results of laboratory tests. As medicine continues to discover and seeks to treat silent diseases in symptomless bodies, the boundaries between health and illness become uncertain and blurred (Vuckovic & Nichter 1997) and people's capacity to retain confidence in their health and consequently, also, themselves is hard to sustain.

Fear of becoming dependent on medicines is a recurrent theme throughout the literature (Conrad 1985; Grime & Pollock 2003; Townsend, Hunt & Wyke 2003). This concern often relates more directly to a concern about psychological, rather than physiological, dependency. Grime and Pollock (2003) describe the uncertainty and ambivalence of many patients towards taking antidepressants, especially in the long term. Even where treatment had been readily accepted at the outset, perspectives could change as patients became uncertain about how much of their recovery was 'genuine', or an artefact of treatment. They came to doubt their capacity to cope without antidepressants, especially if faced with stressful experiences in future and consequently, also, their personal competence and sense of agency. Some respondents sought to test the efficacy of their treatment, and the robustness of themselves, by stopping early. Others continued to take antidepressants, albeit reluctantly, because they were uncertain about their ability to cope without them, and resisted putting this to the test. Attitudes to antidepressant treatment shifted and changed over time, often in ways that patients could not anticipate in advance. However, once established, negative perceptions of the self as vulnerable and unable to cope without chemical support were very difficult to override.

Patients' responses to treatment and associated medicine-taking behaviour are framed by cultural norms that tablet taking in general, and psychotropic medication in particular, is undesirable and to be resisted. At the same time, the consumption of medicines continues to rise, and to extend to an increasing number of conditions or even risk factors, such as raised blood pressure or cholesterol levels (Kawachi & Conrad 1996). Vuckovic and Nichter (1997) point to the paradox of the increased choice and availability of medicines as a personal technology to enhance health and wellbeing and seeming to foster agency, while actually increasing social and personal dependency on professional medicine. People's resistance to taking medicines, and their concerns about the risks and harms that might result from doing so are set against the highly aggressive marketing of medicines as commodities which are indispensable not just to treat disease, but also to promote wellbeing and even to withstand the stresses of a pressurised world. Medicines such as antacids, analgesics and even antidepressants promise to enhance people's capacity to overcome the pain and discomfort which would otherwise impede their ability to remain socially and economically productive. They help people save time and fulfil their obligations. The convenience and promise of medicines sits uneasily alongside the rhetoric of self-reliance and social and personal concern about their potential hazards and toxicity (Davis 1997; Williams & Calnan 1996).

The population also has to contend with further contradictions within the health system and medical establishment, which seek to contain rising prescribing costs and rationalise medicine taking and prescribing (Audit Commission 1994). From a medical perspective, high rates of non-compliance are regarded as irrational, harmful and wasteful, but patients are also castigated for making inappropriate demands on the system, for example in relation to use of antibiotics and proton pump inhibitors (Grime, Pollock & Blenkinsopp 2001; Little *et al.* 1997; Little *et al.* 2004; Weiss & Fitzpatrick 1997). In response to these conflicting messages patients tread a difficult path between balancing the benefits and harms of pharmaceuticals, trust in professionals and distrust of medicines, resistance to treatment and acceptance of expert authority, a desire for autonomy and doubts about personal competence. An awareness of this background and context is necessary for professionals to understand and respond sensitively to patients' concerns about treatments, and their medicine-taking behaviour. It is within the context of this background of concern and ambivalence about medicines that patients approach and assess their consultations with doctors.

References

Adams S, Pill R and Jones A (1997) Medication, chronic illness and identity: the perspective of people with asthma. *Social Science and Medicine.* **45**: 189–201.

Anderson R and Bury M (1988) *Living with Chronic Illness: the experience of patients and their families.* Unwin Hyman, London.

Arluke A (1980) Judging drugs: patients' conceptions of therapeutic efficacy in the treatment of arthritis. *Human Organization.* **39**: 84–7.

Asscher AW, Parr GD and Whitmarsh VB (1995) Towards the safer use of medicines. *BMJ.* **311**(14 October): 1003–5.

Audit Commission (1994) *A Prescription for Improvement: towards more rational prescribing in general practice.* HMSO, London.

Backett K (1992) Taboos and excesses: lay moralities in middle class families. *Sociology of Health and Illness.* **14**: 255–74.

Benson J and Britten N (2002) Patients' decisions about whether or not to take antihypertensive drugs: qualitative study. *BMJ.* **325**(19 October): 873.

Blaxter M (1982) *Mothers and Daughters: a three generation study of health attitudes and behaviour.* Heinneman Educational Books, London.

Blaxter M (1983) The causes of disease: women talking. *Social Science and Medicine.* **17**(2): 59–69.

Blaxter M (1993) Why do the victims blame themselves? In: A Radley (ed.) *Worlds of Illness: biographical and cultural perspectives on health and disease.* Routledge, London, pp. 124–42.

Blumhagen D (1980) Hyper-tension: a folk illness with a medical name. *Culture Medicine and Psychiatry.* **4**: 197–227.

Briceland LL (2000) *Medication Errors: an expose of the problem.* Medscape Pharmacists. http://www.medscape.com/viewarticle/408559 (accessed 28 September 2005).

Britten N (1994) Patients' Ideas About Medicines: a qualitative study in a general practice consultation. *British Journal of General Practice.* **44**: 465–8.

Britten N, Stevenson F, Gafaranga J, Barry C and Bradley C (2004) The expression of aversion to medicines in general practice consultations. *Social Science and Medicine.* **59**: 1495–1503.

Bury M (1982) Chronic illness as biographical disruption. *Sociology of Health and Illness.* **4**: 167–82.

Bury M (2001) Illness narrative, fact or fiction? *Sociology of Health and Illness.* **23**: 263–85.

Campbell P, Cobb A and Darton K (1998) *Psychiatric Drugs: users' experiences and current policy and practice.* Mind Publications, London.

Charmaz K (1983) Loss of self: a fundamental form of suffering in the chronically ill. *Sociology of Health and Illness.* **5**(2): 169–93.

Chetley A (1990) *A Healthy Business? World health and the pharmaceutical industry.* Zed Books, London.

Cobb A, Darton K and Kiran J (2001) *Mind's Yellow Card for Reporting Drug Side Effects: a report of users' experiences.* Mind Publications, London.

Cohen D, McCubbin M, Collin J and Perodeau G (2001) Medications as social phenomena. *Health.* **5**(4): 441–69.

Coleman B (2003) Producing an information leaflet to help patients access high quality drug information on the Internet: a local study. *Health Information and Libraries Journal.* **20**: 160–71.

Conrad P (1985) The meaning of medications: another look at compliance. *Social Science and Medicine.* **20**: 29–37.

Conrad P (1997) The noncompliant patient in search of autonomy. *Hastings Centre Report.* August: 15–17.

Cornwell J (1985) *Hard Earned Lives: accounts of health and illness from East London.* Tavistock, London.

Corry P, Hogman G and Sandamas G (2002) *That's Just Typical.* NSF, London.

Crawford R (1984) A cultural account of health: control, release and the social body. In: JB McKinley (ed.) *Issues in the Political Economy of Health Care.* Tavistock, London.

Davis P (1997) *Managing Medicines.* Open University Press, Buckingham.

Day JC, Kinderman P and Benthall RP (1998) A comparison of patients' and prescribers' beliefs about neuroleptic side-effects: prevalence, distress and causation. *Acta Psychiatrica Scandinavica.* **97**: 93–7.

de Joncheere K, Haaijer-Ruskamp FM, Rietveld AH and Dukes MNG (2003) Scope of the problem. In: MNG Dukes *et al.* (eds) *Drugs and Money: prices, affordability and cost containment* (7e). IOS Press/WHO, Amsterdam, pp. 7–13.

Donovan J (1995) Patient decision making, the missing ingredient in compliance research. *International Journal of Technology Assessment in Health Care.* **11**: 443–55.

Donovan J and Blake D (1992) Patient non-compliance: deviance or reasoned decision-making? *Social Science and Medicine.* **35**(5): 507–13.

Dowell J and Hudson H (1997) A qualitative study of medication-taking behaviour. *Family Practice.* **14**(5): 369–75.

Dunnell K and Cartwright A (1972) *Medicine Takers: prescribers and hoarders.* Routledge and Kegan Paul, London.

Elwyn G and Gwyn R (1999) Stories we hear and stories we tell: analysing talk in clinical practice. *BMJ.* **318**(16 January): 186–8.

Evans-Pritchard EE (1937) *Witchcraft, Oracles and Magic Among the Azande.* Oxford University Press, Oxford.

Fallsberg M (1991) *Reflections on Medicines and Medication: a qualitative analysis among people on long term drug regimens.* Linkoping University, Linkoping.

Frank A (1995) *The Wounded Storyteller: body, illness, and ethics.* University of Chicago Press, Chicago.

Good B (1994) *Medicine, Rationality, and Experience: an anthropological perspective.* Cambridge University Press, Cambridge.

Grime J and Pollock K (2003) Patients' ambivalence about taking antidepressants: a qualitative study. *Pharmaceutical Journal.* **271**(11): October, 516–19.

Grime J, Pollock K and Blenkinsopp A (2001) Proton pump inhibitors: perspectives of patients and their GPs. *British Journal of General Practice.* **51**: 703–11.

Hannay D (1979) *The Symptom Iceberg: a study of community health.* Routledge and Kegan Paul, London.

Haynes RB (1979) Strategies to improve compliance with referrals, appointments and prescribed medical regimes. In: RB Haynes and DL Sackett (eds) *Compliance in Health Care.* Johns Hopkins University Press, Baltimore.

Heath I (2003) A wolf in sheep's clothing: a critical look at the ethics of drug taking. *BMJ.* **327**(11 October): 856–8.

Herzlich C (1973) *Health and Illness: a social psychological analysis.* Academic Press, London.

Hogman G and Sandamas G (2000) *A Question of Choice.* NSF, London.

Hunter MS and Britten N (1997) Decision making and hormone replacement therapy: a qualitative analysis. *Social Science and Medicine.* **45**: 1541–8.

Hyden, L-C (1997) Illness and narrative. *Sociology of Health and Illness.* **19**(1): 48–69.

Hyden, L-C and Peolsson M (2002) Pain gestures: the orchestration of speech and body gestures. *Health.* **6**(3): 325–45.

Illich I (1975) *Medical Nemesis.* Caldar and Boyars, London.

Institute of Medicine (2000) *To Err is Human: building a safer health system.* National Academy Press.

Kagawa-Singer M (1993) Redefining health: living with cancer. *Social Science and Medicine.* **37**: 295–304.

Kangas I (2001) Making sense of depression: perceptions of melancholia in lay narratives. *Health.* **5**(1): 76–92.

Kawachi I and Conrad P (1996) Medicalization and the pharmacological treatment of blood pressure. In: P Davis (ed.) *Contested Ground: public purpose and private interest in the regulation of prescription drugs.* Oxford University Press, Oxford, pp. 26–41.

Kleinman A (1988) *The Illness Narratives: suffering, healing and the human condition.* Basic Books, United States.

Launer J (2002) *Narrative-based Primary Care: a practical guide.* Radcliffe Medical Press, Oxford.

Lewis DK, Robinson J and Wilkinson E (2003) Factors involved in deciding to start preventive treatment: qualitative study of clinicians' and lay people's attitudes. *BMJ.* **327**(11 October): 841.

Lisper L, Isacson D, Sjoden, P-O and Bingefors K (1997) Medicated hypertensive patients' views and experience of information and communication concerning antihypertensive drugs. *Patient Education and Counselling.* **32**: 147–55.

Little P, Dorward M, Warner G, Stephens K, Senior J and Moore M (2004) Importance of patient pressure and perceived pressure and perceived medical need for investigations, referral, and prescribing in primary care: nested observational study. *BMJ.* **328**: 444.

Little P, Williamson I, Warner G, Gantley M and Kinmonth A L (1997) Open randomised trial of prescribing strategies in managing sore throat. *BMJ.* **314**: 722–7.

Misselbrook D (2001) *Thinking About Patients.* Petroc Press, Newbury.

Morgan M (1996) Perceptions and use of anti-hypertensive drugs among cultural groups. In: S Williams and M Calnan (eds) *Modern Medicine: lay perspectives and experiences.* UCL Press, London, pp. 95–116.

Morris DB (1998) *Illness and Culture in the Postmodern Age.* University of California Press, Berkeley.

Payer L (1989) *Medicine and Culture: notions of health and sickness in Britain, the US, France and Germany.* Victor Gollanz Ltd, London.

Pellegrino ED (1976) Prescribing and drug ingestion: symbols and substances. *Drug Intelligence and Clinical Pharmacy.* **10**: 624–30.

Petit-Zeman S, Sandamas G and Hogman G (2001) *Doesn't It Make You Sick? Side Effects of Medicine and Physical Health Concerns of People With Severe Mental Illness.* NSF, London.

Pill R and Stott N (1982) Concepts of illness causation and responsibility: some preliminary data from a sample of working class mothers. *Social Science and Medicine.* **16**: 43–52.

Pirmohamed M, James S, Meakin S, Green C, Scott AK, Walley TJ, Farrar K, Park BK and Breckenridge AM (2004) Adverse drug reactions as cause of admission to hospital: prospective analysis of 18 820 patients. *BMJ.* **329**(3 July): 15–19.

Pollock K (1993) Attitude of mind as a means of resisting illness. In: A Radley (ed.) *Worlds of Illness: biographical and cultural perspectives on health and disease.* Routledge, London.

Pound P, Britten N, Morgan M, Yardley L, Pope C, Daker-White G and Campbell R (2005) Resisting medicines. *Social Science and Medicine.* **61**(1): 133–55.

Radley A (1993) The role of metaphor in adjustment to chronic illness. In: A Radley (ed.)

Worlds of Illness: biographical and cultural perspectives on health and disease. Routledge, London, pp. 109–23.

Rogers A, Day JC, Williams B, Randall F, Wood P, Healy D and Benthall RP (1998) The meaning and management of neuroleptic medication: a study of patients with a diagnosis of schizophrenia. *Social Science and Medicine*. **47**: 1313–23.

Rogers A and Pilgrim D (1993) Service users' views of psychiatric treatments. *Sociology of Health and Illness*. **15**(5): 612–31.

Sachs L (1995) Is there a pathology of prevention? The implications of visualizing the invisible in screening programmes. *Culture Medicine and Psychiatry*. **19**: 503–25.

Sandars J and Esmail A (2003) The frequency and nature of medical error in primary care: understanding the diversity across studies. *Family Practice*. **20**(3): 231–6.

Starland B (2001) New paradigms for quality in primary care. *British Journal of General Practice*. **51**: 303–9.

Stevenson F, Wallance G, Rivers P and Gerrett D (2000) 'It's the best of two evils': a study of patients' perceived information needs about oral steroids for asthma. *Health Expectations*. **2**: 185–94.

Stimson G and Webb B (1975) *Going to See the Doctor: the consultation process in general practice*. Routledge and Kegan Paul, London.

Strauss A and Corbin J (1998) *Basics of Qualitative Research: techniques and procedures for developing grounded theory*. Sage Publications, Thousand Oaks.

Townsend A, Hunt K and Wyke S (2003) Managing multiple morbidity in mid-life: a qualitative study of attitudes to drug use. *BMJ*. **327**(11 October): 837.

Vuckovic N and Nichter M (1997) Changing patterns of pharmaceutical practice in the United States. *Social Science and Medicine*. **44**(9): 1285–302.

Wadsworth M, Butterfield W and Blaney R (1971) *Health and Sickness: the choice of treatment*. Tavistock, London.

Wadsworth M and Robinson D (1976) *Studies in Everyday Medical Life*. Martin Robertson, London.

Weiss M and Fitzpatrick R (1997) Challenges to medicine: the case of prescribing. *Sociology of Health and Illness*. **19**(3): 297–327.

West P (1976) The physician and the management of childhood epilepsy. In: M Wadsworth and D Robinson (eds) *Studies in Everyday Medical Life*. Martin Robertson, London.

Williams G (1984) The genesis of chronic illness: narrative reconstruction. *Sociology of Health and Illness*. **6**: 175.

Williams G (1993) Chronic illness and the pursuit of virtue in everyday life. In: A Radley (ed.) *Worlds of Illness: biographical and cultural perspectives on health and disease*. Routledge, London, pp. 92–108.

Williams R (1983) Concepts of health: an analysis of lay logic. *Sociology*. **17**: 185–205.

Williams S and Calnan M (1996) Modern medicine and the lay populace in late modernity. In: S Williams and M Calnan (eds) *Modern Medicine: lay perspectives and experience*. UCL Press, London, pp. 256–64.

Wright M (2000) The old problem of adherence: research on treatment adherence and its relevance for HIV/AIDS. *Aids Care*. **12**: 703–10.

Zola IK (1975) Medicine as an institution of social control. In: C Cox and A Mead (eds) *A Sociology of Medical Practice*. Collier-MacMillan, London, pp. 170–246.

Zola IK (1977) Healthism and disabling medicalization. In: I Illich *et al.* (eds) *Disabling Professions*. Marion Boyars Publishers, London, pp. 41–68.

Chapter Five

The doctor–patient relationship

The doctor–patient relationship is framed at any given time by wider social and cultural constraints, and particularly the dominant mode of production of medical knowledge, and the association between the medical profession and the state. The currently entrenched high social status and authority of doctors is a relatively recent development. Medical practitioners in pre-scientific times were a disparate and relatively lowly group. Jewson (1976) has characterised practice around the end of the eighteenth century as 'Bedside Medicine'. Physicians worked directly for affluent patrons of the upper and emerging middle classes. Diagnosis and treatment of the ills afflicting the patient, or 'sick man', were based on close observation of his external form, and attentive listening to accounts of his subjective experience. Within the holistic cosmology of the time illness was taken to be an expression of personal disorder and misalignment rather than the manifestation of discrete, arbitrary and regularly recurring disease entities. The patient played a central role in commissioning the service, constituting the illness and evaluating the efficacy of treatment.

The development of scientific enquiry following the Enlightenment combined with factors deriving from the social and economic transformations of the industrial revolution to produce fertile ground for the expansion of medical expertise and social status. Rapid urbanisation and widespread squalor led to high rates of disease and ill health. Initially in Paris, and subsequently throughout the rest of Europe, the establishment of the charity hospitals provided a concentration of patients which was ideal for the practice of scientific medicine, and also a stimulus to the development of statistical inference and the emerging discipline of epidemiology. As scientific medicine progressed, the medical gaze moved beyond the patient's external form to penetrate his interior body and to explore the signs and processes of pathology in individual organs and tissues. As the patient's testimony became increasingly redundant to the processes of diagnosis and treatment of disease, his subjective experience of illness and distress came increasingly to be disregarded (Armstrong 1995; Jewson 1976).

Hospital patients in the nineteenth century occupied a socially inferior position to the physicians who learned so much from the passive bodies presented for their scrutiny. May and Mead (1998) observe that this social distance may be one source of the public deference to medical authority that persists to the present day. Continuing private patronage of a greatly expanded middle class increased the demand for medical services and also provided economic security for the rapidly increasing population of physicians. Increased collegiate organisation among practitioners established a basis for professionalisation, a process fostered by the state in the course of extending its involvement and responsibility firstly for public health and later also the health of individual citizens. In 1858 the Medical Act granted a legal monopoly for approved doctors to practise medicine, and allowed the profession to select, train and regulate the conduct of its members (Jewson 1976; May & Mead 1998; Porter 1997).

The social status of doctors also rose through the association of medicine with the authority of science. The third stage of Jewson's typology, laboratory medicine, developed through the latter decades of the nineteenth century and into the twentieth. The focus of production of medical knowledge moved outside the patient altogether, to the investigation of individual cells and biochemical processes. Confirmation and diagnosis of disease could now take place independently of the patient, and even in a laboratory far removed from his presence. Personal testimony concerning the symptoms and experience of illness became redundant. At this point, the patient loses his voice altogether. Whatever he has to say can be disregarded in the face of definitive evidence adduced from expert appraisal of the scientific tests and markers of disease. The consequences of largely writing out the patient from the process of diagnosis and evaluation of medical intervention have had a critical impact on consultations between patients and health professionals, which will be taken up for discussion in subsequent chapters.

Porter (1997) describes medical practice in the second half of the nineteenth century as an age of 'therapeutic nihilism' in which treatment efficacy lagged far behind the great progress being made in accurately diagnosing and understanding disease. In compensation, the 'patient as person' movement developed as a strand of practice in the opening decades of the twentieth century. In the absence of effective treatment, the importance of the doctor–patient relationship was emphasised, along with the need to provide psychosocial support and the therapeutic benefits that could derive from this. However, even to the extent that physicians may have been sensitive to the need to provide patients with encouragement and a sense of *feeling* better, this was applied in a markedly paternalistic and authoritarian manner (Armstrong 1982; Cassidy 1938). The normative construction of the patient as passive, deferential and obedient to medical authority was expressed in the hugely influential model of the sick role put forward by the sociologist Talcott Parsons in the 1950s (Parsons 1958). Incumbency of the sick role involved two rights and two obligations: the patient was not held to be responsible for his illness, and was entitled to (temporary) exemption from normal roles and responsibilities. In return, he had to actively engage in the effort to recover, and to this end to seek and comply with medical advice and treatment. In exercising judgement about the nature and legitimacy of illness the doctor was in a position of considerable power in determining individual access to a wide range of resources, including treatment and economic and social benefits.

Armstrong (1982) charts the change in professional representations of the patient from the early to the middle decades of the twentieth century: the 'patient as person' was rediscovered from the end of the interwar period (Armstrong 1982). More effective drugs were developed in response to changing disease profiles. Increasing numbers of people were prescribed long-term complex therapeutic regimes to treat chronic disease. Alongside the realisation that many failed to comply with these, attention focused on understanding the reasons for such apparently irrational behaviour and developing effective techniques for improving adherence. Even though these mainly involved straightforwardly manipulative attempts to change behaviour, the effort to engage patients' cooperation in increasing compliance entailed an awareness of the individual as a responsive agent, rather than a purely passive receptacle for pathology. Attention shifted to the importance and quality of communication between doctor and patient as a determinant of therapeutic efficacy (Ley 1979; Ley & Spelman 1967).

Early epidemiological surveys revealed the high prevalence of different forms of ill health throughout the population (Koos 1954). Together with the influence of Freudian theories of psychoanalysis and the new discipline of psychology, the perceived ubiquity of pathology eroded the boundaries between health and illness, normality and abnormality. Illness, particularly mental illness, was reconfigured as a continuum, rather than a dichotomous category, affecting everyone to a degree, at certain times. The patient's subjective experience emerged as a principal site of pathology and became a primary focus of interest. The profile of the social medicine movement was boosted by the work of Michael Balint in the 1950s. Balint (1957) came to general practice having trained in psychoanalysis. He stressed the importance of empathy between doctor and patient, and the need for professional awareness and manipulation of patients' experience of psychosocial difficulties that often underlay the consultation. The quality of the relationship between doctor and patient was viewed as an important source of therapeutic efficacy in its own right. The skilful deployment of the doctor's 'apostolic function' was actively promoted as a means of helping the substantial proportion of patients in primary care whose reasons for consulting were now recognised to relate at least partly to functional disorders and/or problems which are psychosocial in origin (Kleinman & Sung 1979).

At the same time, and also from within psychiatry, Szasz and Hollender (1956) put forward a tripartite model of the doctor–patient relationship. 'Activity-passivity' denoted a type of consultation controlled and dominated by the doctor, with the patient merely a passive and cooperative subject. 'Guidance-cooperation' applied to consultations where the patient played a more active role, but was strongly influenced by medical judgement. The third model, involving 'mutual participation', much more nearly approached an equal partnership between doctor and patient. The potential contribution and *interests* of the patient were recognised, and a redrawing of the boundaries of power and influence within the consultation was placed on the agenda. Szasz and Hollender considered that each model had a role to play, and that particular context would determine which was the most appropriate. Nevertheless, they noted that empirically the 'mutual participation' model was rare, and did not envisage that it would achieve a more prominent position in the medical culture of the future.

A further influential model originating within psychiatry was proposed by Engel in the 1970s (Engel 1977; Engel 1980). Engel argued that the biomedical model, with its narrow focus on organic disease, had outlived its usefulness. The biopsychosocial model was proposed as a means of uniting the disparate fields of mental and physical disorder. It was necessary to acknowledge the psychosocial components of illness, and their contribution to the manifestation and experience of all forms of disease, mental or physical. The biopsychosocial model was sensitive to the ways in which the biomedical model neglected the patient. It incorporated a holistic perspective of the individual's suffering and experience of dis-ease. However, just as Balint and his followers had been concerned to emphasise the distinctive expertise of the general practitioner, Engel aimed to boost the status and acceptability of psychiatry as a legitimate medical speciality. Thus, the biopsychosocial itself was framed within a discourse of interprofessional competition and territoriality. The patient might find himself viewed more compassionately, but his role remained one of passive acquiescence. The physician retained his expert status in diagnosing illness and interpreting its causes, albeit from a more humanistic 'biopsychosocial' perspective.

The models outlined above proposed a realignment of the doctor–patient relationship but did not threaten to undermine professional authority, or the status and credibility of biomedicine as a social practice. However, from the 1960s onwards, medicine has been subject to a series of sustained and more challenging critiques, originating from within the profession as well as outside it. The realisation of great technological advancement and therapeutic efficacy was accompanied by diverse forms of social and professional resistance as the power of medicine to harm as well as heal became evident. Concern was raised about the iatrogenic effects of medical treatment, graphically portrayed by the effects of the thalidomide tragedy in the late 1960s. Revelations about the inappropriate use and widespread addiction of patients to tranquillisers, prescribed to relieve relatively minor symptoms of anxiety and distress, provoked widespread disquiet about the misapplication of medical technology (Gabe & Bury 1996). The malign capacity of medicine to pathologise large areas of everyday life and experience and subject them to professional sureveillance and regulation was recognised and resisted (Boston Women's Health Collective 1976; Conrad 1981; Illich 1975; Kawachi & Conrad 1996; Williams & Calnan 1996b; Zola 1975; Zola 1977). The natural childbirth and antipsychiatry movements were particularly effective in focusing attention on the extent to which medicine was overreaching itself in appropriating the authority to make judgements about moral issues which belonged more properly to personal and social arenas. For example, expert medical opinion was used to establish the boundaries between the mad and the bad, the deviant and the sick, to control access to procedures such as abortion and assisted conception, and to set down standards for how individuals should lead their lives, under the guise of promoting 'healthy' behaviour (Conrad 1981; Zola 1975; Zola 1977). New disease states, requiring medical diagnosis and intervention, were created out of biological experiences and conditions hitherto regarded as natural and normal, such as menstruation, the menopause, pregnancy and even the process of ageing (Kawachi & Conrad 1996). Other, disvalued, forms of behaviour, such as overeating, disruptive behaviour and drug and alcohol abuse, were labelled as pathological and requiring treatment (Conrad 1981; Double 2002). An increasing range of 'risk factors' have been identified, such as raised blood pressure and cholesterol levels, being overweight or, increasingly, just being old, for which long-term medical surveillance and pre-emptive treatment is advocated (Kawachi & Conrad 1996).

Even in the 1970s, Illich was writing not just of clinical but also of cultural iatrogenesis by which perceived dependence on medicine robs individuals of their capacity to cope independently with pain and suffering as an inevitable aspect of life. Social iatrogenesis occurs through the institutional dominance of biomedicine, which precludes realistic choice or access to alternative forms of care (Illich 1975). Freidson spearheaded a trenchant critique of professional dominance (Freidson 1970; Illich 1977; McNight 1977; Zola 1975) which viewed the extension of medical jurisdiction as a means of fostering professional power and self-interest. Professional expertise involved the *application* of knowledge which was, invariably, ideologically filtered. The cloak of scientific neutrality masked the moral saturation of medical judgement. As professional interventions penetrate more deeply into all aspects of people's lives, their capacity for autonomy and self-determination becomes eroded. Medical dominance feeds off the social dependency generated by the demand it induces for its services. In acquiring the capacity both to define needs, as well as evaluate the benefits that patients supposedly derive from its interventions, medicine effectively derails personal autonomy and disables citizenship (Freidson 1970; Illich 1977; McNight 1977; Zola 1975; Zola 1977).

The professional dominance critique developed mainly within the social sciences. However, another attack on orthodox medicine, and particularly psychiatry, was led from within medicine itself, and also originated in the 1960s. The antipsychiatry movement did not just aim to liberalise and humanise psychiatric practice. Rather it questioned its entire basis. Psychiatric diagnoses were viewed as instruments of personal oppression and social control. Szasz (1970, 1972) rejected the claim that psychiatric disorders constituted organic disease states: psychiatric diagnoses were *metaphors* for disease. The reification of such metaphors and the application of psychiatric labels to what are fundamentally experiences and problems of living, rather than pathological states, serves to further the aggrandisement of the psychiatric profession as state agents of social control. A further critique of the repressive functions of psychiatry was given in Laing and Esterson's analysis of schizophrenia as a coping strategy originating in dysfunctional social and specifically family relationships, rather than organic disease. The complicity of psychiatry in medicalising personal distress was a manifestation of its symbiotic relationship with the state for which it functioned as a means of containing non-conformity and maladjustment. The theories of Laing and Esterson (Laing 1960; Laing & Esterson 1970) were widely popularised in the 1960s, and a powerful stimulus to social scepticism about the legitimacy of psychiatry.

According to labelling theory, mental illness is not so much a condition or attribute of the person, as a product of social responses to certain forms of culturally deviant or disapproved behaviour, especially in weak or vulnerable social groups or categories (Becker 1963; Scheff 1966). In applying highly stigmatising labels to individuals manifesting certain kinds of disvalued experiences and behaviour, psychiatric diagnoses function as a means of containing social disruption and reinforcing conformity. Once applied, stigmatising labels cannot be removed, and not only are the affected individuals viewed in terms of the social stereotypes associated with the labels, they come to internalise these, and conform to the stereotypes associated with them. A celebrated study by Rosenhan (1973) revealed the importance of context and social expectations, as well as the power of professionals, in institutional settings. Eight sane researchers managed to gain admission to a number of North American mental hospitals solely on the basis of saying they had heard voices in their head. This was the only manifestation of reported or behavioural normality they gave throughout the entire experiment. All but one was given a diagnosis of schizophrenia. Once attached to the diagnosis, the pseudopatients found it very difficult to get the hospital staff to recognise their normality, and let them out of hospital. They were discharged an average of 19 days later (range from 7 to 52 days) and even then with a diagnosis of 'schizophrenia in remission', rather than a restitution of their sanity. Labelling theorists varied in the extent to which they saw mental illness as actually generated by social definitions and responses, or shaped by them. However, their work drew attention to the coercive and arbitrary nature of psychiatric practice.

The antipsychiatry movement of the 1960s was part of a culture of protest involving resistance to many things: war, racism, medicalisation, environmental pollution, social inequality and patriarchy, among others (Kelleher, Gabe & Williams 1994). It was a time of intense preoccupation with the relationship between the individual and the state, and the assertion of autonomy as a moral principle. Although the force of social protest subsided subsequently, the anti-psychiatry movement boosted the development of the user movement, strands of which have remained actively critical of psychiatric practice (Campbell 1996; Crossley 1998; Crossley & Crossley 2001; Read & Reynolds 1996). Although dwarfed by the established authority of the conventional biomedical model, a critique of psychiatry has also continued from within the profession (Boyle 1990; Breggin 1993; Ingleby 1981; Johnstone 2000; Kutchins & Kirk 1999; Newnes, Holmes & Dunn 1999; Newnes, Holmes & Dunn 2001; Treacher & Baruch 1981). At the present time it is particularly associated with the work of the postpsychiatry group (Bracken & Thomas 2001; Double 2002; Faulkener & Thomas 2002).

A further critique of biomedicine grew out of an increasing awareness that health inequalities remained extensive even in affluent industrial societies. In European countries such as Britain this was so in spite of an established and comprehensive state welfare system. Such inequalities were determined much more by social and economic factors than individual behaviour or medical intervention (Jacobsen, Smith & Whitehead 1991; Townsend, Davidson & White-head 1990; Townsend, Phillimore & Beattie 1988; Wilkinson 1996). McKeown (1979) had demonstrated that public health measures such as the widespread provision of clean water and sanitation followed by rising living standards and improved nutrition throughout the nineteenth and early twentieth centuries had had a much greater impact in improving the population's health and reducing mortality from infectious disease than any biomedical interventions available at the time. However, the introduction of really effective remedies such as the sulpha drugs and penicillin from the 1930s, and the rapid development of new drugs and surgical procedures thereafter, contributed to the conviction that modern medicine was essential to the treatment of disease and restoration of health. This is not to deny the very considerable achievements of medical technology or the benefits it can deliver. However, modern medicine has been extremely successful in convincing itself and an often very willing public that its attainments have been extraordinary, when historically its contribution has been overrated.

In Britain the power of doctors was reinforced by the establishment of the NHS in 1948. This provided a comprehensive health service, funded from taxation, giving the whole population entitlement to healthcare according to need, and free at point of delivery. Widely regarded as the 'jewel in the crown' of the state welfare system, the NHS undoubtedly benefited the general population, whilst at the same time considerably furthering the interests of the medical profession. From its inception, the NHS represented a compromise. Both general practitioners and hospital physicians were granted a very considerable degree of professional and clinical autonomy, confirming the power of the medical profession and dominance of the existing professional hierarchy. Reflecting the interests of the doctors who controlled decisions about treatment, the major proportion of healthcare resources were allocated to high technology, high prestige but very specialised hospital-based healthcare. This has made it difficult to rationalise the system, or to redirect resources to greater areas of need among the general population, the so-called 'Cinderella services' such as those for the old, and mentally ill or disabled, or into public health and preventive health measures which could potentially deliver greater health gains for a substantially greater proportion of the population (Allsop 1995; Baggott 1994; Ham 1992; Jones 1994).

From the outset, political management of the NHS has been concerned to contain escalating costs of healthcare, achieve a fairer distribution of resources, and impose greater accountability on clinical practice. However, little impact was made until the reforms of the Thatcher government introduced an industry-based managerial culture following the Griffiths report of 1983 (DHSS 1983) and the establishment of an internal market in healthcare following the NHS and Community Care Act of 1990. Patient consumerism was encouraged as a means of furthering an ideological commitment to individual choice as well as raising standards in healthcare (Hunter 1994). From this point onwards, the health service has been subject to continuing change and modification aimed at increasing efficiency and cost-effectiveness, raising standards and evaluating clinical perform-ance. The Labour government has subsequently continued the policy of turning the NHS into a patient-centred service, responsive to patient preferences and appraisal, and offering choice as well as quality of service (Appleby, Harrison & Devlin 2003; Coulter 2002a; Coulter 2002b; Department of Health 1996, 1998, 1999, 2000, 2001a, 2001b, 2002, 2003; Rycroft-Malone *et al.* 2001).

Health professionals are now subject to an unprecedented degree of appraisal and evaluation. These include processes of clinical governance, prescribing guidelines, monitoring of prescribing rates and patterns and fixed prescribing budgets. Since the introduction of the GMS contract for general practitioners in April 2004, remuneration has been linked more extensively to achievement of specific performance targets for example, in relation to immunisation pro-grammes and screening, prescribing of statins, and waiting lists and times for appointment.

Greater patient involvement and also responsibility for healthcare is encour-aged through the commitment to developing 'partnerships' between professionals and service users. Increasing patient involvement in this way is seen as intrinsically desirable, in rendering publicly funded services more democratic, responsive and transparent, and also recognising and enabling individual auton-omy through the exercise of informed choice. Concordance slots easily into this model of patient-centred healthcare. Patient participation in healthcare is also a politically attractive strategy in providing an additional source of external accountability. Patient choice can be a convenient political foil for monitoring and directing professional performance. Increased representation of patients at all levels of health service organisation, for example, through the Patient Forums of individual Primary Care Trusts, Citizens' Juries and Citizens' Councils set up by NICE, are means of potentially involving the public directly in the process of clinical governance (Appleby, Harrison & Devlin 2003).

Increasing regulation and surveillance of medical work over the past two decades has prompted consideration of the impact on clinical autonomy and the extent to which health professionals have been subject to a processes of proletarianisation and deprofessionalisation (Armstrong 2003; Harrison & Dowsell 2002; Lupton 1994; Lupton 1997; McKinley & Stoeckle 1988; Weiss & Fitzpatrick 1997; Williams & Calnan 1996a). The proletarianisation thesis asserts that there has been a substantive reconfiguration in the relationship between professionals and the state. Increased regulation and bureaucratic accountability has curtailed the clinical autonomy which was at the heart of traditional professionalism. Doctors now occupy the same position in the labour market as other workers, and have been divested of the essential privileges they once possessed over the control of their work. As we have seen in Chapter 3, the movement to evidence-based medicine has been interpreted as a means of professional readjustment in order to retain the right to continuing self-regulation, standard setting and evaluation of professional practice. Against this, however, it has been argued that the adoption of evidence-based practice has merely resulted in a restratification of the profession, in which the main body of doctors are now subject to direction from a specialist elite who are themselves constrained to implement policy objectives as directed by the state (Armstrong 2003; Harrison & Dowsell 2002; Weiss & Fitzpatrick 1997; Williams & Calnan 1996a).

The deprofessionalisation thesis proposes that the narrowing of the competence gap between doctors and patients has substantially undermined the authority of medicine (Harrison & Dowsell 2002; Lupton 1997; Weiss & Fitzpatrick 1997; Williams & Calnan 1996a). A wide range of modern media – particularly the internet – has massively expanded lay access to specialist information and eroded the monopoly of knowledge which was formerly an important basis of professional power. In addition, the public has acquired a greater political sophistication and wider social awareness of the hazards of medicine and of the contested nature of scientific knowledge. Scepticism and distrust of expert knowledge is a characteristic feature of late modern societies (Harrison & Dowsell 2002; Lupton 1997; Weiss & Fitzpatrick 1997; Williams & Popay 1994; Williams & Calnan 1996a). Increasingly consumer-oriented patients have become more assertive and less deferential to medical authority.

Available evidence suggests that doctors are more concerned about the impact of trends towards deprofessionalisation rather than protelarianisation of medical practice. Several studies have reported their GP respondents to be fairly sanguine about the increased bureaucratic accountability and greater managerial control they recognised to be affecting their work (Harrison & Dowsell 2002; Lupton 1997; Weiss & Fitzpatrick 1997). However, Lupton and Weiss and Fitzpatrick reported that their respondents were much more concerned about the adverse effects of what they perceived to be an increase in demanding and 'consumerist' patients, and felt these to constitute a greater threat to their clinical autonomy than increased state regulation. This is so, despite the fact that there is very little evidence, throughout an extensive literature, that patients are deviating to any great extent from their traditional role of passive deference to health professionals in medical consultations (Barry *et al.* 2000; Britten 1995; Britten *et al.* 2000; Cox *et al.* 2004; Gillespie, Florin & Gillam 2002; Hogg 1999; Lupton 1997; Makoul, Arntson & Schofield 1995; McKinstry & McKee 2000; Weiss & Fitzpatrick 1997).

It seems that there is a considerable distance between professional perceptions or expectations of patient behaviour in medical consultations, and the reality of what actually happens. It is extraordinary that, in spite of the seismic social, economic and professional changes to which medicine has been subject over the past several decades, as outlined above, there continues to be such a gulf between the rhetoric of patient-centred medicine, and its practice (Coulter 2002b; Rycroft-Malone *et al.* 2001). How is it possible that, notwithstanding several decades of sustained pressure, the substance of the medical consultation, and the enactment of the traditional roles of patient and doctor, remain basically unchanged? This question is taken up for consideration in the following chapter.

References

Allsop J (1995) *Health Policy and the NHS: towards 2000* (2e). Longman, Harlow.

Appleby J, Harrison A and Devlin N (2003) *What is the Real Cost of More Patient Choice?* King's Fund, London.

Armstrong D (1982) The doctor–patient relationship 1930–1980. In: P Wright and A Treacher (eds) *The Problem of Medical Knowledge*. Edinburgh University Press, Edinburgh, pp. 109–21.

Armstrong D (1995) The rise of surveillance medicine. *Sociology of Health and Illness.* **17**(3): 393–404.

Armstrong D (2003) Clinical autonomy, individual and collective: the problem of changing doctors' behaviour. *Social Science and Medicine.* **55**(10): 1771–7.

Baggott R (1994) *Health and Health Care in Britain*. Macmillan Press, London.

Balint M (1957) *The Doctor, His Patient, and the Illness*. Pitman Medical, London.

Barry C, Bradley C, Britten N, Stevenson F and Barber N (2000) Patients' unvoiced agendas in general practice consultations. *BMJ.* **320**: 1246–50.

Becker H (1963) *Outsiders: studies in the sociology of deviance*. Free Press, New York.

Boston Women's Health Collective (1976) *Our Bodies, Ourselves*. Revised edn. Simon and Schuster, New York.

Boyle M (1990) *Schizophrenia: a scientific delusion?* Routledge, London.

Bracken P and Thomas P (2001) Postpsychiatry: a new direction for mental health. *BMJ.* **322**(24 March): 724–7.

Breggin P (1993) *Toxic Psychiatry, Drugs and Electroconvulsive Therapy: the truth and better alternatives*. HarperCollins, London.

Britten N (1995) Patients' demands for prescriptions in primary care. *BMJ.* **310**(29 April): 1084–5.

Britten N, Stevenson F, Barry C, Barber N and Bradley C (2000) Misunderstanding in prescribing decisions in general practice: a qualitative study. *BMJ.* **320**: 484–8.

Campbell P (1996) The history of the user movement in the United Kingdom. In: T Heller *et al.* (eds) *Mental Health Matters: a reader*. Macmillan/Open University, London, pp. 218–26.

Cassidy M (1938) Doctor and patient. *The Lancet.* **January 15**: 175–9.

Conrad P (1981) On the medicalization of deviance and social control. In: D Ingleby (ed.) *Critical Psychiatry*. Penguin, Harmondsworth, pp. 102–19.

Coulter A (2002a) After Bristol: putting patients at the centre. *BMJ.* **324**(16 March): 648–51.

Coulter A (2002b) *The Autonomous Patient: ending paternalism in medical care*. The Nuffield Trust, London.

Cox K, Stevenson F, Britten N and Dundar Y (2004) *A Systematic Review of Communication Between Patients and Health Care Professionals about Medicine-taking and Prescribing*. Medicines Partnership, London.

Crossley ML and Crossley N (2001) 'Patient' voices, social movements and the habitus; how psychiatric survivors 'speak out'. *Social Science and Medicine.* **52**(10): 1377–94.

Crossley N (1998) RD Laing and the British anti-psychiatry movement: a socio-historical analysis. *Social Science and Medicine.* **47**(7): 877–89.

Department of Health (1996) *Patient Partnership: building a collaborative strategy.* Department of Health, National Health Service Executive, London.

Department of Health (1998) *In the Public Interest: developing a strategy for public participation in the NHS.* Department of Health NHS Executive, London.

Department of Health (1999) *Patient and Public Involvement in the New NHS.* Department of Health, London.

Department of Health (2000) *The NHS Plan: a plan for investment, a plan for reform.* Department of Health, London.

Department of Health (2001a) *Involving Patients and the Public in Healthcare: a discussion document.* Department of Health, London.

Department of Health (2001b) *The Expert Patient: a new approach to chronic disease management for the 21st century.* Department of Health, London.

Department of Health (2002) *Learning from Bristol: the DH response to the report of the public inquiry into children's heart surgery at the Bristol Royal Infirmary 1984–1995.* Department of Health, London.

Department of Health (2003) *Building on the Best: choice, responsiveness and equity in the NHS.* Department of Health, London.

DHSS (1983) *NHS Management Inquiry (The Griffiths Management Report).* DHSS, London.

Double D (2002) The limits of psychiatry. *BMJ.* **324**: 900–4.

Engel GL (1977) The need for a new medical model: a challenge for biomedicine. *Science.* **196** (4286): 129–36.

Engel GL (1980) The clinical application of the Biopsychosocial Model. *Americal Journal of Psychiatry.* **137**(5): 535–44.

Faulkener A and Thomas P (2002) User-led research and evidence-based medicine. *British Journal of Psychiatry.* **180**: 1–3.

Freidson E (1970) *Professional Dominance.* Atherton, New York.

Gabe J and Bury M (1996) Anxious times: the benzodiazepine controversy and the fracturing of expert authority. In: P Davis (ed.) *Contested Ground: public purpose and private interest in the regulation of prescription drugs.* Oxford University Press, Oxford, pp. 42–56.

Gillespie R, Florin D and Gillam S (2002) *Changing Relationship: findings from the patient involvement project.* King's Fund, London, Executive summary.

Ham C (1992) *Health Policy in Britain: the politics and organisation of the national health service* (3e). Macmillan Press, London.

Harrison S and Dowsell G (2002) Autonomy and bureaucratic accountability in primary care: what English general practitioners say. *Sociology of Health and Illness.* **24**(2): 208–26.

Hogg C (1999) *Patients, Power and Politics: from patients to citizens.* Sage Publications, London.

Hunter DJ (1994) From tribalism to corporatism: the managerial challenge to medical dominance. In: J Gabe, D Kelleher and G Williams (eds) *Challenging Medicine.* Routledge, London, pp. 1–22.

Illich I (1975) *Medical Nemesis.* Caldar and Boyars, London.

Illich I (1977) Disabling Professions. In: I Illich *et al.* (eds) *Disabling Professions.* Marion Boyars Publishers, London, pp. 11–39.

Ingleby D (1981) *Critical Psychiatry: the politics of mental health.* Penguin, Harmondsworth.

Jacobsen B, Smith A and Whitehead M (1991) *The Nation's Health, A Strategy for the 1990s: a report from an Independent Multidisciplinary Committee.* King Edward's Hospital Fund for London, London.

Jewson ND (1976) The disappearance of the sick man from medical cosmology 1770–1870. *Sociology.* **10**: 225–44.

Johnstone L (2000) *Users and Abusers of Psychiatry.* Routledge, London.

Jones L (1994) *The Social Context of Health and Health Work.* Macmillan Press, London .

Kawachi I and Conrad P (1996) Medicalization and the pharmacological treatment of blood pressure. In: P Davis (ed.) *Contested Ground, Public Purpose and Private Interest in the Regulation of Prescription Drugs.* Oxford University Press, Oxford, pp. 26–41.

Kelleher D, Gabe J and Williams G (1994) Understanding medical dominance in the modern world. In: J Gabe, D Kelleher and G Williams (eds) *Challenging Medicine.* Routledge, London, pp. xi–xxix.

Kleinman A and Sung LH (1979) Why do indigenous practitioners successfully heal? *Social Science and Medicine.* **13B**: 7–26.

Koos EL (1954) *The Health of Regionville: what the people thought and did about it.* Columbia University Press, New York.

Kutchins H and Kirk SA (1999) *Making us Crazy: DMS – the psychiatric bible and the creation of mental disorders.* Constable, London.

Laing RD (1960) *The Divided Self.* Tavistock Publications, London.

Laing RD and Esterson A (1970) *Sanity, Madness and the Family: families of schizophrenics.* Pelican Books, London.

Ley P (1979) Improving clinical communication: effects of altering doctor behaviour. In: D Oborne, M Gruneberg and J Eiser (eds) *Research in Psychology and Medicine.* Academic Press, London.

Ley P and Spelman MS (1967) *Communicating with the Patient.* Staples Press, London.

Lupton D (1994) *Medicine as Culture: illness, disease and the body in western societies.* Sage Publications, London.

Lupton D (1997) Doctors on the medical profession. *Sociology of Health and Illness.* **19**(4): 480–97.

Makoul G, Arntson P and Schofield T (1995) Health promotion in primary care: physician–patient communication and decision making about prescription medications. *Social Science and Medicine.* **41**(9): 1241–54.

May C and Mead N (1998) Patient-centredness: A history. In: L Frith and C Dowrick (eds) *Ethical Issues in General Practice: Uncertainty and Responsibility.* Routledge, London, pp. 76–90.

McKeown T (1979) *The Role of Medicine: dream, mirage, or nemesis?* Blackwell, Oxford.

McKinley JB and Stoeckle JD (1988) Corporatization and the social transformation of doctoring. *International Journal of Health Services.* **18**(2): 191–205.

McKinstry A and McKee M (2000) Do patients wish to be involved in decision making in the consultation? A cross sectional survey with video vignettes. *BMJ.* **321**: 867–71.

McNight J (1977) Professionalized service and disabling help. In: I Illich *et al.* (eds) *Disabling Professions.* Marion Boyars Publishers, London, pp. 69–92.

Newnes C, Holmes G and Dunn C (1999) *This is Madness: a critical look at psychiatry and the future of mental health services.* PCCS Books, Ross-on-Wye.

Newnes C, Holmes G and Dunn C (2001) *This is Madness Too: critical perspectives on mental health services.* PCCS Books, Ross-on-Wye.

Parsons T (1958) Definitions of health and illness in the light of the American values and social structure. In: E Jaco (ed.) *Patients, Physicians and Illness.* Free Press, New York.

Porter R (1997) *The Greatest Benefit to Mankind: a medical history of humanity from antiquity to the present.* HarperCollins, London.

Read J and Reynolds J (1996) *Speaking Our Minds: an anthology of personal experiences of mental distress and its consequences.* The Open University, Milton Keynes.

Rosenhan DL (1973) On being sane in insane places. *Science.* **179**: 250–8.

Rycroft-Malone J, Latter S, Yerrell P and Shaw D (2001) Consumerism in health care: the case of medication information. *Journal of Nursing Management.* **9**: 221–30.

Scheff T (1966) *Being Mentally Ill: a sociological theory.* Weidenfield and Nicolson, London.

Szasz TS (1970) *The Manufacture of Madness.* Harper and Row, New York.

Szasz TS (1972) *The Myth of Mental Illness: foundations of a theory of personal conduct.* Paladin, London.

Szasz TS and Hollender MH (1956) A contribution to the philosophy of medicine: the basic models of the doctor–patient relationship. *Archives of Internal Medicine.* **97**: 585–92.

Townsend P, Davidson N and Whitehead M (1990) *Inequalities in Health: the Black Report and the health divide.* Penguin, Harmondsworth.

Townsend P, Phillimore P and Beattie A (1988) *Health and Deprivation: inequality and the North.* Routledge, London.

Treacher A and Baruch G (1981) Towards a critical history of the psychiatric profession. In: D Ingleby (ed.) *Critical Psychiatry.* Penguin, Harmondsworth, pp. 120–49.

Weiss M and Fitzpatrick R (1997) Challenges to medicine: the case of prescribing. *Sociology of Health and Illness.* **19**(3): 297–327.

Wilkinson R (1996) *Unhealthy Societies.* Routledge, London.

Williams G and Popay J (1994) Lay knowledge and the privilege of experience. In: J Gabe, D Kelleher and G Williams (eds) *Challenging Medicine.* Routledge, London, pp. 118–39.

Williams S and Calnan M (1996a) Modern medicine and the lay populace: theoretical perspectives and methodological issues. In: S Williams and M Calnan (eds) *Modern Medicine: lay perspectives and experiences.* UCL Press, London, pp. 2–25.

Williams S and Calnan M (1996b) Modern medicine and the lay populace in late modernity. In: S Williams and M Calnan (eds) *Modern Medicine: lay perspectives and experience.* UCL Press, London, pp. 256–64.

Zola IK (1975) Medicine as an institution of social control. In: C Cox and A Mead (eds) *A Sociology of Medical Practice.* Collier-Macmillan, London, pp. 170–246.

Zola IK (1977) Healthism and disabling medicalization. In: I Illich *et al.* (eds) *Disabling Professions.* Marion Boyars Publishers, London, pp. 41–68.

Chapter Six

The medical consultation

<blockquote>

Box 6.1

The patient is continually open to new information about his illness and use of medicines from friends and others. He will possibly be continually reassessing the consultation, the doctor's action, and the prescribed medicine. The patient is repeatedly faced with the problem of whether he is doing the right thing with regard to his health.

Stimson (1974)*

</blockquote>

Contemporary research has confirmed the persisting empirical rarity of the patient participation model of the consultation. Indeed, this has been a recurrent theme from the early studies of the patient perspective in the 1970s and 1980s through to the present day. Stimson and Webb (1975) first introduced the patient's perspective of the medical encounter. Their study revealed the contrast between the passive and deferential demeanour of patients during the consultation, and the critical appraisal they brought to bear on this afterwards (Box 6.1). Byrne and Long (1976) found that the overwhelming majority of the 2500 consultations they analysed were dominated by the doctor. Attempts to elicit patient ideas or concerns, or to invite patients' active participation in the interview were rare. Their argument that medical care and health outcomes would be improved by encouraging patients to play an active role in managing their healthcare was taken forward in the 1980s by Tuckett et al. (1985).

Tuckett et al.'s study extended understanding of the mechanisms underlying good communication and the consequences of participants' lack of understanding of the different perspectives each party brought to the medical encounter. It also highlighted the extent to which patients contributed to the success of the consultation, both as a social and a therapeutic encounter. The study involved 16 GPs, and was based on tape recordings of 1302 of their consultations, and detailed follow-up interviews with a sample of 328 patients. There are some striking similarities between this study and that of Byrne and Long. The investigators found major shortcomings in the amount and quality of information given by GPs to their patients and concluded that these doctors were rather ineffective communicators. Virtually without exception, the GPs displayed a complete lack of interest in, or awareness of, patients' own ideas and understanding of the illness. Consequently, no attempt was made to relate their medical explanations to the individual explanatory models of the disorder held by the patients. The doctors made little effort to establish how their advice and information had been received by patients, or whether they had understood what they had been told. The researchers observed that the GPs were uneasy or intolerant of patients' endeavours to express their own ideas or concerns about their illness. In over half of the consultations the doctors attempted to evade or suppress patients' expression of ideas. In only one in five of the consultations did doctors appear even to tolerate patients' disclosure of their ideas by listening without interrupting. The minority of patients who persisted in taking a more active role in the consultation pursued a risky strategy. They were more likely to have their views explored, and to receive fuller explanations from the doctors. However, they were also more likely to provoke an overt expression of tension in the consultation. Ordinarily, both doctor and patient collaborated to avoid situations where conflict or hostility was overt. An important reason for patients' reluctance to play a more active part in the consultation was their fear of antagonising the doctor, and the risk of jeopardising their future care. Another common reason for not asking questions was the concern about pressure of time, and an awareness of feeling hurried in the consultation.

Contrary to the widespread assumptions about patients' limited capacity for recalling information, Tuckett *et al.* found that most patients (90%) were able to recall accurately the key points made by their doctors during the consultations. Most were also able to attribute a correct meaning to what they had been told. This capacity of patients to reproduce the *sense* of what they had been told, rather than recall the specific terms in which it was conveyed, was also a finding of Donovan's study of arthritis patients (Donovan 1995). It seems that when attention is directed to the construction of meaning, patients are revealed as much more competent than the conventional 'recall of information' studies would suggest (Ley 1982).

Paradoxically, there appeared to be no association between the doctor's capacity to give a clear and full explanation and the patients' capacity to achieve an adequate understanding of what they had been told. Some respondents misunderstood what seemed to be clear and straightforward accounts by their doctors. Others made perfect sense of confusing or inadequate advice. What seemed to matter most was not the clarity of the information given by the doctor, but the patient's ability to interpret this in the light of the prior knowledge, experience and expectations he brought to the consultation. Patients had often diagnosed the problem, and anticipated their GP's response, correctly. In this case, where both parties were operating with a similar explanatory framework of the illness, the patients were able to 'fill in' and make sense of the gaps or lack of clarity in the information given to them by their doctors. In situations of ambiguity or uncertainty, however, where patients had formulated a different explanatory model of the illness from that of their doctors, they were likely to misinterpret or forget even clear statements of information, because they lacked the interpretive framework necessary to make sense of it (see also Punamaki & Kokko 1995a). Because the doctors had no interest in patients' ideas or emotional concerns, and rarely made any effort to check that the patient had correctly understood what he had been told, they remained unaware of the extent to which misunderstandings had occurred. They also failed to realise the importance of the contributory work which many patients were making to the success of the consultation. Patients who did not recall or accept their doctor's advice were less likely to follow it, and conversely.

Tuckett *et al*. argued that there was a need for a substantial change in doctors' perceptions of their role, and the ways they related to patients. In characterising the consultation as a 'meeting between experts', Tuckett was not attributing the same kind of specialist technical expertise to patients that was held by doctors. The point is rather that the patient brings a unique knowledge of how his illness is experienced, and situates this within a particular set of concerns and aspirations. The aim of medical consultations should be to help patients arrive at informed decisions about how best to manage their health problems, rather than the unilateral production of medical judgements about how this should be done.

In justifying the argument that a change in the traditional doctor–patient relationship was needed, Tuckett anticipated that the continuation of several trends would render such a development both increasingly appropriate and likely. A compelling reason for facilitating patient choice is that it is patients who have to live with the consequences of illness and treatment. This has particular salience in relation to the often intrusive nature of modern therapies, as well as the uncertainty relating to their efficacy and ratio of benefit to harm (Starland 2001). A second justification for developing more patient-centred consultations is the therapeutic benefit that patients can derive from a supportive relationship with their doctors. As the incidence of chronic degenerative conditions continues to rise among the ageing populations of the industrialised nations, the provision of information, reassurance and understanding becomes an important part of therapy in its own right. It may even constitute the only therapy (Kleinman 1988). Patient motivation is particularly important in the management of chronic illness. Patients who remain uncommitted to the treatment suggested by their doctors are less likely to follow their advice (Britten *et al*. 2000; Korsch & Negrete 1972; Tuckett *et al*. 1985). Finally, Tuckett anticipated that patients would continue to become increasingly well informed as part of the general trend towards increased consumerism in society. As this happened, they would become more inclined to assert their preferences in the consultation, and doctors would become more approachable and accepting of such an approach.

Tuckett *et al*.'s study was carried out nearly 20 years ago and, consequently, its relevance to the present day might be questioned. However, in addition to the quality of the investigation, the results of this study are significant because they point to the amount of change that has *not* occurred (Rycroft-Malone *et al*. 2001) in the intervening period. As Tuckett anticipated, patients have continued to become better informed about matters relating to health and illness. The burden of chronic disease continues to increase, and doubts (medical and public) about the effectiveness and net benefit of many treatments have acquired a higher profile (Asscher, Parr & Whitmarsh 1995; Barry *et al*. 1988; Department of Health 2002; Dieppe *et al*. 2004; Frankel, Ebrahim & Davey Smith 2000; Institute of Medicine 2000; Kawachi & Conrad 1996; Medawar 1997; Petit-Zeman, Sandamas & Hogman 2001; Pirmohamed *et al*. 2004; Wennberg *et al*. 1993). Information technology has transformed the transfer and distribution of knowledge in society. In addition, the development of patient-centred medicine and active partnerships between patients and professionals have become central planks in government health policy (Department of Health 1991, 1996, 1998a, 1998b, 1999, 2000, 2001a, 2001b, 2003). Nevertheless, there has been surprisingly little substantive change in the nature of the doctor–patient relationship or the structure of the consultation (Barry *et al*. 2000; Britten *et al*. 2000; Butler, Campion & Cox 1992;

Coulter 2002; Cox *et al.* 2004; Ehrich 2003; Elwyn, Edwards & Kinnersley 1999; Kettunen *et al.* 2001; Ley 1997; Little *et al.* 2001; Makoul, Arntson & Schofield 1995; Meredith 1993; Ohtaki, Ohtaki & Fetters 2003; Punamaki & Kokko 1995b; Roter *et al.* 1997; Roter 2000; Rycroft-Malone *et al.* 2001; Schwartz, Soumeris & Ajorn 1989; Stevenson *et al.* 2000; Tate 2003; Wiles & Higgins 1996). Tuckett's analysis remains as relevant today as it was in the mid 1980s. There has been some change in research terminology (see below) and some reduction in the social distance between doctors and patients, and probably also an increased informality in their interrelations. But these are superficial changes: the 'bureaucratic format' of the medical consultation depicted by Strong in another classic study of the 1970s has survived through the decades substantially intact (Strong 1979).

Strong's analysis of the bureaucratic format was derived from observation of a Scottish paediatric clinic, but as he suggested, it is widely applicable throughout the state health service. Its focus is on the organisational context in which individual action occurs, rather than the qualities or behaviours of individual actors. The consultation is characterised by routinisation, brevity, impersonality and politeness. The patient role is one of passive deference to professional expertise, with little scope for active intervention. The consultation is controlled by the professional, proceeding at the doctor's pace, and leaving little time for patients to pause for thought, reflect on what had been said, or reframe a question. Such encounters are not conducive to the discussion of patients' fears and concerns about their condition, and patients are generally reluctant to raise such issues. The surface manifestation of routinised detachment and civility frequently overlays the experience of tension and unease.

A considerable body of more recent research confirms the continuing professional domination of medical encounters. These studies have consistently described the limited extent of patient participation in the consultation and the lack of professional awareness and elicitation of patient concerns and understandings of illness which underlie the decision to consult (Barry *et al.* 2000; Butler *et al.* 1998; Cockburn & Pitt 1997; Coulter 1997; Cromarty 1996; Elwyn, Edwards & Kinnersley 1999; Guadagnoli & Ward 1998; Punamaki & Kokko 1995a; Roter *et al.* 1997; Stevenson *et al.* 2000). Barry *et al.* (2000) carried out a detailed examination of 35 general practice consultations using a similar methodology to that employed by Tuckett *et al.* (1985). This revealed that patients brought a range of issues, concerns and expectations to the consultation (agendas), many of which were never aired or addressed. Every patient had at least one agenda item and most had at least five. However, only four of the 35 patients in the study voiced all items of their agendas in the consultations. The most common concerns related to worries about diagnosis, expectations of the future, side effects of drugs and the impact of illness on patients' social circumstances. The most frequently raised agenda items related to symptoms, diagnosis and requests for prescriptions. Patients were less likely to raise emotional or psychosocial concerns during the consultation. These unvoiced agendas were related to misunderstandings between doctor and patient and to 'problem outcomes' which included patients being issued with unwanted prescriptions, or deciding not to follow the treatment advised. The researchers identified 14 categories of misunderstanding between doctors and patients relating specifically to the taking of medicines, which occurred in 28 of the 35 consultations. In every case these misunderstandings were related to the lack of patient participation in the consultation. For example, patients often did not express their preferences either for or against receiving a prescription. In the absence of any evidence to the contrary, doctors made assumptions about what patients thought or were expecting from the consultation, and had no source of feedback to alert them to the inaccuracies of their perceptions. In particular, the doctors lacked awareness of the significance – or even the existence – of patients' ideas in influencing their illness behaviour and willingness to follow medical advice (Britten *et al.* 2000).

An accumulating body of research over the last 30 years has established that medical consultations continue to exhibit a structured asymmetry characterised by the passive and overtly deferential demeanour of the patient and interactional dominance by the doctor. This is in spite of considerable encouragement for the development of a more 'consumerist' orientation among patients, and the practice of more 'patient-centred' medicine by professionals. It is not entirely clear why it has proved so difficult to engineer a change in the substance of medical culture, rather than the rhetoric. However, it seems that to a great extent both patients and professionals remain locked within the constraints of the bureaucratic format depicted by Strong (1979), and the associated etiquette which governs behaviour within the consultation.

Although routine encounters for professionals, medical consultations are often difficult, complex and emotionally charged events for patients (Bloor & Horobin 1975; Freidson 1975; Silverman 1987; Stimson & Webb 1975; Strong 1979; Tuckett *et al.* 1985; Werner & Malterud 2003; Zola 1981). The decision to seek professional advice can be difficult. Patients often express anxiety about having made a misjudgement and consulted inappropriately for trivial or insubstantial conditions (Cornford 1998; Cromarty 1996; Kadam *et al.* 2001; Neal, Heywood & Morley 2000; Pattenden *et al.* 2002; Pollock & Grime 2002; Punamaki & Kokko 1995a; Punamaki & Kokko 1995b). Concern about getting this wrong can lead to potentially grave consequences. Pattenden *et al.* (2002) investigated patients' reasons for delay in seeking help after having a heart attack. Respondents took as long to respond to the experience of a second episode as they had done over the first. In addition to being reluctant to admit the need for help, they did not want to cause trouble, especially if this involved imposing on the system outside normal working hours. Anxiety and embarrassment at the prospect of being wrong in their interpretation of symptoms were also reasons for the delay in seeking help. The problematic nature of the decision to consult, and patient's concern to establish that they have legitimate grounds for doing so, reflect a norm that professional help should only be sought in case of extreme or genuine need. This points to a tension between patients, professionals and the healthcare system, in terms of setting boundaries of entitlement and access.

Patient concerns about consulting inappropriately are validated by the negative professional stereotypes of their behaviour articulated in the 'patient defect model'. Patient expectations and 'demand' for services are construed as inappropriate and excessive (Bradley 1992a; Bradley 1992b; Rogers, Hassell & Nikolaas 1999; Weiss *et al.* 1996; Weiss & Fitzpatrick 1997). Professional irritation at being confronted by 'trivia' derives from the norm that physical illness rather than psychosocial distress constitutes the proper grounds for medical consultation (Cartwright & Anderson 1981; Dowrick *et al.* 1996). A number of studies have described how doctors struggle to deal with patients who repeatedly present with vague, ill-defined and seemingly intractable symptoms and problems. The crux of the matter involves the incommensurability of the conflicting explanatory models which patients and doctors bring to bear in interpreting these inchoate manifestations and experiences. Patients often reject the professional ascription of psychosocial causation in favour of more 'legitimate' and less stigmatising organic models of pathology (Chew-Graham *et al.* 2002; Chew-Graham & May 1999; Dixon-Woods & Critchley 1999; May *et al.* 2004; Raine *et al.* 2004; Rogers, May & Oliver 2001; Werner & Malterud 2003).

The difficulties posed by people who attend frequently with enduring, unresolvable, and frequently psychosocial problems are well expressed by terms such as 'heartsink', 'fat file' or even 'hateful' patient (Bellon & Fernandez-Asensio 2002; Butler & Evans 1999; Dixon-Woods & Critchley 1999; Dowrick 1992; Gerrard & Riddell 1988; Groves 1978; Mathers, Jones & Hannay 1995; O'Dowd 1988). Mindful of these stereotypes, patients strive to avoid them (Coyle 1999; Neal, Heywood & Morley 2000). Patients and doctors alike seem to operate with very similar models of 'good' and 'bad' patients (Bastian 2003; Cohen & Britten 2003; Dixon-Woods & Critchley 1999; Kettunen *et al.* 2001; McKevitt & Morgan 1997; Neal, Heywood & Morley 2000; Stokes, Dixon-Woods & McKinley 2003, 2004). 'Good' patients are cooperative, polite, respectful, consult appropriately and considerately, accept professional judgement, follow medical advice, and are not openly critical or challenging of their doctors. Although patients generally work hard to fulfil the role of 'good' patient, they do not always succeed. In an account of frequent general practice attenders, Neal described the tension for patients in not wanting to consult inappropriately and the need to allay their anxieties about what was wrong. Respondents were aware that their doctors regarded them to be overly demanding and, as such, a nuisance. They were apprehensive about incurring professional disapproval and attracting pejorative labels such as hypochondriac. These frequent attenders tried to consult considerately and, in their terms, appropriately. They only consulted when they felt it was necessary for them to do so, and considered that this was often because their doctor had initiated a further appointment for a check-up, or in order to review medication (Neal, Heywood & Morley 2000). A powerful justification for patients' concern to behave well, and not to antagonise their doctors, is the very real risk that they may find themselves struck off his list (Stokes, Dixon-Woods & McKinley 2003, 2004).

Detailed analysis of communication between doctors and patients reveals the tightly controlled rules of the interactional order governing the conduct of medical consultations (Heritage 1997; Maynard 1991; Robinson 2001; Taylor & White 2000; ten Have 1991). Participants endeavour to establish their personal competence and moral adequacy through the successful presentation of face (Bloor & Horobin 1975; Ehrich 2003; Kettunen *et al.* 2001; Lambert 1995a; Lambert 1995b; Robins & Wolf 1988; Stimson & Webb 1975; Werner & Malterud 2003). Goffman defined face as 'the positive social value a person effectively claims for himself by the line others assume he has taken during a particular contact' (1972: 5). Face is, effectively, the expression of personal identity and self-esteem, and consequently carries a strong emotional charge. Loss of face entails embarrassment or even humiliation. Face cannot be sustained independently, but is achieved (or undermined) in interaction with others, i.e. it is a social accomplishment, depending on mutual cooperation and assent. Consequently, it is usually in the individual's best interests to assist in maintaining the face of other participants in an interaction, as, under ordinary circumstances, he can rely on their support in preserving his own. The desire to maintain face is a fundamental principle of social interaction. This is conventionally achieved by the observation of social courtesy and politeness, as constituted in the 'ceremonial order' (Strong 1979).

Brown and Levinson differentiated positive and negative face and associated forms of politeness (Brown & Levinson 1978). Negative politeness works to maintain the boundaries of personal autonomy through non-imposition on others. It is characterised by formality, emotional distance and routinisation. Positive politeness asserts a commonality of identity and interests between participants, and hence their intrinsic desirability. Positive politeness functions as a 'social accelerator', inviting or demonstrating intimacy between participants. However, unwarranted assumptions of mutuality may cause offence. Consequently, positive politeness is a risky strategy and its use tends to be restricted.

Negative politeness is exemplified in the formal and distancing routines characteristic of interaction between strangers and in 'institutional talk' (Heritage 1997) in which there may often be a status disparity between participants. Brown and Levinson (1978) observe that a primary strategy of negative politeness is to circumvent the display of asymmetric power relationships, which are strongly disvalued in Western cultures. Any suggestion of command or compulsion between two speakers is highly threatening to face. Participants who have sufficiently high social status may disregard the face of others if they feel they have no need to save their own. However, in ordinary circumstances, the conventions of courtesy and politeness prevail. The display of power and status differentials is highly stylised and muted by the routines and strategies of negative politeness.

Medical consultations are difficult encounters to bring off successfully, being intrinsically face-threatening to both participants. This accounts for the formal politeness and affective neutrality which characterises the 'bureaucratic' routine described by Strong as a mechanism for containing conflict and emotional tension. However, consultations are particularly threatening for patients. In making demands on their doctors through the disclosure of problems (particularly emotional distress), and the assertion of need, patients immediately place themselves in a vulnerable and discreditable position. The act of consulting itself entails relinquishing autonomy. The requirement to disclose highly personal, sensitive – perhaps overtly embarrassing – information to the doctor heightens this disadvantage, and underlines the structured asymmetry in the relationship between patients and practitioners. Aside from the intrinsic anxiety involved in the experience of illness, consultations contain moral hazard for the patient. Negative attributions of incompetence in consulting behaviour and self-care, as well as the implication of lifestyle factors and personal responsibility for ill health are highly discreditable. The difficult and socially disvalued status of 'patient' is well illustrated by McKevitt and Morgan in their account of GPs' personal responses to becoming ill and their resistance to occupying the sick role (McKevitt & Morgan 1997). Illness was viewed as a manifestation of weakness and vulnerability, and inappropriate for doctors. It was associated with feelings of shame, dependency, and compromised autonomy.

The negative imagery associated with the role of patient provides at least a partial explanation for the great concern which people feel about consulting appropriately, not wasting professional time and performing adequately as a 'good' patient. In addition, patients depend on professionals for access to resources and entitlements which can have very significant implications for their wellbeing, but over which they have not direct leverage. These extend far beyond treatment and referrals, to include sickness and other benefits, legitimation of sick leave, insurance and mortgage status, and even occupational fitness (Maseide 1991; Maynard 1991). It is not surprising that patient behaviour should be characterised by deference and politeness and the desire to retain the doctor's goodwill.

Doctors, also, have a desire to maintain face – of themselves, as well as their patients – as a demonstration of professional and personal competence. Like patients, they work hard to avoid the overt expression of conflict in the consultation and to protect the therapeutic relationship. Coleman *et al.* describe the selective processes and contexts in which GPs chose to raise the subject of smoking with patients in consultations, in order to avoid giving offence (Coleman, Murphy & Cheater 2000). Much clinically inappropriate prescribing has been attributed to doctors' desire to please their patients and invest in their longer term relationship, even though they were often mistaken in their assumptions about what patients wanted, or were expecting from the consultation (Bradley 1992a; Britten 1995; Britten 2004; Freeman & Sweeney 2001; Rees Jones *et al.* 2004; Tomlin, Humphrey & Rogers 1999; Veldhuis, Wigersma & Okkes 1998; Weiss & Scott 1997).

Negative politeness and the professional concern to maintain face serves also as a means of coping with the demands of professional uncertainty and anxiety. Nevertheless, it is clear that it is patients who bear the brunt of the discomfort associated with medical consultations, and who are most vulnerable to loss of face. The role of patient is negatively valued and interactionally subordinate to that of the professional. The structured asymmetry of the consultation is reproduced through well established strategies and conversational routines which operate substantially to the patient's disadvantage (Maynard 1991; ten Have 1991). Professionals control the interaction in monopolising initiatives such as turn taking, asking questions, determining the ratio of closed to open enquiries, and withholding information.

Beckman *et al.* found that the majority of doctors interrupted the patient's opening statement of concerns after an average of 18 seconds of speech, thus preventing a complete account of the presenting agenda for the consultation. Only one out of 51 patients was subsequently able to return to this at a later stage in the consultation. As a result it is likely that the consultation focused on only some of the patient's concerns, and not necessarily the most important ones (Beckman & Frankel 1984). This study was replicated 12 years later, with substantially similar findings (Marvel *et al.* 1999). Less than a third (74:28%) of patients succeeded in completing their opening statement of concern. The doctors interrupted and redirected opening statements after a mean of 23.1 seconds. On average, patients took only 26 seconds to state their full concerns, and consultations in which this was accomplished lasted only six seconds longer than those in which the patient's opening agenda was interrupted.

Robinson's analysis revealed the differential impact of doctors' interactional strategies in closing the consultation on patient opportunities to raise additional concerns. Given the normative expectation that each consultation should deal with only one problem, it is difficult for patients to find a suitable 'window of opportunity' for the presentation of additional issues (Campion & Langdon 2004; Robinson 2001). In a study of depression in general practice, Pollock and Grime describe how some of their respondents self-consciously rationed the problems and questions they presented, planning to introduce these over a series of visits, in order not to overburden a single consultation (Pollock & Grime 2002).

Conversation analysts have stressed the extent to which structured asymmetry in consultations is interactively achieved. It is a product of the communicative exchange and even collaboration between patients and professionals, rather than the gross imposition of institutional power or constraints of external organisational structure (Maynard 1991; ten Have 1991). In reproducing the expected roles of passive patient and proactive doctor, participants reinforce and validate the norms of the encounter: they behave in what they have come to view as the expected and appropriate manner. This complicity of patients in contributing to the structured asymmetry of the consultation is well illustrated by Kettunen *et al.*'s analysis of 38 counselling consultations between Finnish patients and nurses (Kettunen *et al.* 2001). Patient 'taciturnity' was a noted feature of half of these encounters. Respondents were keen to present themselves as 'good', cooperative and considerate patients. They tried to help the nurses by not wasting time – even passing up the opportunity to talk at greater length in order to achieve this. The interactional dominance of the nurses was facilitated by patients' politeness, restricted speech and the use of face-saving devices such as self-deprecating humour and tentativeness. Respondents tended to express their opinions or raise issues in a hesitant and indirect manner, thus allowing nurses to choose whether to respond or disregard. In contrast, nurses interrupted frequently, disregarded patients' speech turns, asked closed questions and often persisted in giving unnecessary information and redundant instructions. The nurses seemed more concerned with pursuing their own agenda and fulfilling institutional and professional objectives than engaging in a meaningful discussion of patients' concerns. Moreover, they seemed oblivious to the extent of the work which patients were undertaking to ensure the success of the encounter. Patient passivity was accepted at face value. From the patients' perspective, however, taciturnity may be a way of saving face, and also a form of self-protection, in maintaining emotional distance and deflecting a more intrusive professional examination of subjectivity.

The respondents in Kettunen *et al.*'s study accepted professional authority and the status of deferential patient. Their taciturnity was offered as cooperation and in some cases, perhaps, a form of self-protection. Silence is a highly effective strategy of negative politeness, since it may be interpreted in many different ways. From a professional perspective, patient passivity may be construed, sometimes correctly, as acceptance, understanding and lack of concern. However, silence may also be used to mask resistance or dissent (Stimson & Webb 1975; Strong 1979; Tuckett *et al.* 1985). Participants usually go to great lengths to avoid the overt expression of conflict or disagreement. Being assertive, even asking questions, may be construed by both professionals and patients as a challenge and a threat to professional face (Cohen & Britten 2003; Kettunen *et al.* 2001; Strong 1979; Tuckett *et al.* 1985). This raises problems about the legitimacy of patient knowledge, and the circumstances under which they may display it. Henwood found that even informed respondents would not divulge their knowledge in the consultation as this would risk transgressing the boundary between patient and expert and thus antagonising the doctor (Henwood *et al.* 2003). Indeed, it is evident that patients may sometimes purposefully present themselves to their doctors in a manner suggestive of greater ignorance than they actually possess (Donovan 1995; Pilnick 1998; Stimson & Webb 1975). Donovan comments that patients sometimes do this deliberately as a means of checking the accuracy and consistency of what different professionals have told them. Well informed and articulate individuals may achieve a degree of interactional equality with professionals, but it seems that this is usually limited (Pilnick 1998). Having consulted an 'expert', patients feel that it is disrespectful, and likely to be construed as a waste of professional time, if they do not at least appear to take the advice that is offered. They may also be reluctant to put their own ideas about illness forward for discussion where these are not perceived to be appropriate topics to raise in a medical consultation (Barry *et al.* 2000). Challenging medical judgement in the consultation risks undermining patients' initial judgement that they need help and puts in question their grounds for consulting: Bloor and Horobin characterise this as the patient 'double bind': they are supposed to have sufficient expertise to judge when medical help is needed, but then to suspend critical appraisal in ceding to professional judgement thereafter (Bloor & Horobin 1975).

Patient passivity in the consultation is frequently in contrast to their behaviour and appraisal outside it. Non-compliance with medical instruction and advice is a classic, and very widespread, manifestation of disagreement and resistance. Stimson and Webb were among the first to describe the ongoing critical evaluation that patients bring to bear on their doctor's performance and the effectiveness and suitability of prescribed treatment. In particular, they describe the use of 'atrocity' stories in which patients are openly critical of professionals and present themselves as taking a much more forcefully proactive part in the consultation than is actually the case. These function as a means of redress against the loss of face and resulting degradation experienced in the role of patient (Stimson & Webb 1975).

In the face of the tensions and difficulties endemic to the consultation, the conventions of the bureaucratic format (Strong 1979) provide interactive devices to stabilise the interaction between patients and doctors, even at the expense of therapeutic outcome. Patients behave, by and large, as they are expected to. In following the rules of the consultation, and adopting the conventional behaviour of passive deference, they often appear to be more accepting of their doctor's definition of the situation, and more committed to following their doctor's advice, than is actually the case. Where patients do not feel comfortable putting forward their concerns, or engaging in active dialogue, professionals have no way of discovering the real agenda underlying the consultation or the extent to which patients' need for information and explanation has been met (Ley 1997). In these circumstances, medical judgements are influenced by expectations and assumptions about what patients think and want, which are often inaccurate. This is one source of inappropriate stereotypes of patients, e.g. that they routinely expect antibiotics for conditions such as respiratory infections for which they are not warranted (Barry *et al.* 2000; Britten 1994; Britten 1995; Britten *et al.* 2000; Britten 2004; Butler *et al.* 1998; Cockburn & Pitt 1997; Little *et al.* 1997; Little *et al.*

2004; Punamaki & Kokko 1995a; Stevenson *et al.* 2000). If patients do not ask questions, it is understandable that doctors might conclude that they have none, or do not require additional information. Patients, on the other hand, tend to expect that relevant information will be provided without their having to ask for it (Kettunen *et al.* 2001).

A common source of conflict and misunderstanding in the consultation has been located in the distinction between *disease* and *illness* (Eisenberg 1978; Kleinman 1986). Disease refers to the occurrence of organic pathology which is the focus of biomedical investigation and treatment. Illness relates to the subjective experience of symptoms and the social context and consequences of their occurrence. Because disease has become so firmly established as the topic of appropriate discourse within the consultation it can be difficult for patients to raise issues relating to their experience of illness, or to feel confident that these are legitimate topics to discuss with their doctors. Thus the language of the consultation may be framed in terms of disease, when the underlying agenda concerns illness. For example, one qualitative study revealed that women may have very different agendas to their GPs concerning the nature of the menopause and the use of HRT. The doctors tended to view menopausal symptoms as pathological, and indicators of disease. The women, on the other hand, considered the menopause to involve a natural process, for which treatment was ordinarily inappropriate (unnatural). Only if symptoms became severe (and so unnatural/pathological) was medical intervention felt to be warranted. In addition, it was found that the women appeared to use HRT for short-term symptomatic relief, rather than for long-term prevention of osteoporosis or heart disease, which is an important medical indication for its use. These features of patients' understanding of menopause help to explain the common reluctance to take HRT for the recommended period of five years: one third of the women took it for no longer than nine months (Hunter & Britten 1997).

Patients may offer concrete signs of disease for discussion, because they feel that it is inappropriate to arrange a consultation purely for information, advice or even reassurance. In particular, they may be reluctant to disclose psychosocial distress, either because they find communicating such experience difficult, or fear the attribution of unwanted and stigmatising diagnostic labels that might result from doing so (Cape & McCullough 1999; Gask *et al.* 2003; Kadam *et al.* 2001). In addition, patients may not consider that it is *necessary* or desirable to consult their GP about depressive or psychosocial symptoms, considering that these may be more appropriately and effectively resolved through other, non-medical, sources of help and support (Cape & McCullough 1999; Murray & Corney 1990; Prior *et al.* 2003). They may also dispute that a diagnosis of depression is appropriate (Cape 2001; Cape & McCullough 1999; Goldberg *et al.* 1998; UMDS MSc in General Practice Teaching Group 1999). It has become a medical truism that depression is routinely undetected and undertreated in general practice (Brown *et al.* 2001; Hale 1997; Montgomery *et al.* 1993a; Montgomery *et al.* 1993b; Thompson *et al.* 1996; Tylee 1995). This observation is frequently accompanied by the view that such omissions lead to markedly increased social and personal costs in the form of more severe and prolonged illness (Hirschfeld *et al.* 1997). However, a number of studies have also reported the 'spontaneous remission' of many cases of depression in general practice, or at least that the course and outcome of depression is no worse among cases that remain undetected and untreated in comparison with patients who receive a diagnosis and treatment with antidepressants (Cape 2001; Cape & McCullough 1999; Dowrick & Buchan 1995; Goldberg *et al.* 1998). Patients' desire to resist the medicalisation of what they regard as fundamentally personal experiences of distress or more general problems of living can thus be viewed as appropriate and legitimate.

A different scenario obtains, however, where patients and doctors disagree about the nature and origins of symptoms which are experienced as concrete but cannot be traced to any physiological cause or malfunction. The phenomenon of 'medically unexplained symptoms' is reported to be widespread, and to constitute a significant source of conflict between patients and professionals (Cape 2001; Cape & McCullough 1999; Goldberg *et al.* 1998; Kroenke 2002; May *et al.* 2004; Wileman, May & Chew-Graham 2002; Woivalin *et al.* 2004). Thus, it can also happen that patients reject a psychosocial explanation of their problems, and struggle to avoid negative stereotypes they feel are associated with these, in opposition to their doctor's judgement (Chew-Graham & May 1999; Dixon-Woods & Critchley 1999; May *et al.* 2004; Werner & Malterud 2003). May *et al.* (2004) describe the difficulties for doctors in relation to patients presenting with back pain and other medically unexplained symptoms. Such diffuse and inde-terminate conditions challenge the epistemological authority of biomedicine, since they cannot be accommodated within the conventional disease paradigm. Doctors' resort to a psychogenic explanation tends to be resisted by patients who reject the negative attribution of supposedly 'neurotic' or 'psychosomatic' disorder. Werner *et al.* (Werner & Malterud 2003; Werner *et al.* 2004) describe a similar response among women suffering from chronic pain, in their efforts to establish the credibility of their experience and protect the integrity of their self-esteem. They worked hard to present themselves as suffering from 'genuinely' somatic disorders, and to avoid the highly stigmatising and resented labels associated with mental instability or psychosomatic illness. For these women, the failure to be believed, or to have the reality and significance of their suffering acknowledged appropriately, was deeply distressing. Werner *et al.* observe that despite its patient-friendly intent, the biopsychosocial model can actually work to their disadvantage in stressing the subjective and psychological dimensions of experiences which patients may prefer to define as organic.

While patients may struggle to resist unwelcome medical categorisation, their doctors struggle to manage cases they regard as frustrating, unrewarding and intractable. Patients presenting with medically unexplained symptoms are par-ticularly face-threatening to doctors, in undermining their authority and profes-sional competence. Wileman, May and Chew-Graham (2002) and Chew-Graham and May (1999) describe doctors' sense of being manipulated by patients presenting with medically unexplained symptoms (MUS) into colluding with inappropriate biomedical explanations of symptoms that they believed to be psychogenic in origin. This route may have been initiated by the instigation of tests, treatment and referrals to satisfy the doctor's concern to eliminate the possibility of organic disease. Where patients are keen to avoid a psychogenic attribution for their problems, doctors may find it difficult to engineer a shift away from biomedical terminology. They then become trapped in what they regard as an unwelcome collusion with patients, in which they contribute, albeit reluc-tantly, to the unwarranted medicalisation of patients' psychosocial distress. The doctors' sense of powerlessness and resentment is mirrored in the accounts of patients describing their struggle for the recognition of their symptoms as genuine and rooted in physiological abnormality (Chew-Graham & May 1999; Salmon, Peters & Stanley 1999; Werner & Malterud 2003; Werner, Widding Isaksen & Malterud 2004). The outcome is a bad relationship between patients and doctors, with very little prospect of an effective therapeutic outcome. Woivalin *et al.* (2004) describe similar findings in relation to GPs' experience and evaluation of MUS patients. Their respondents appeared to adopt a more varied and reflexive approach to managing these, being prepared to shift their explanatory framework in an effort to provide positive support, and also protect their relationship with patients. However, Woivalin notes that her GP respondents did not feel comfortable with the strategy of reinforcing patients' belief in the organic basis of their problems. The doctors recognised that this merely reinforced patients' attachment to what they felt to be an inappropriate explanatory model, and intensified the medicalisation of their problems. Salmon, Peters & Stanley (1999) describe MUS patients' perceptions of their doctors' responses to their presenting complaints in very similar terms to the actual responses reported by Wileman, May and Chew-Graham (2002) and Chew-Graham and May (1999). They identified three categories of perceived responses. Most of their patient respondents felt that their doctors either rejected their explanations of symptoms (as being organically based), or colluded with them, albeit uneasily, by appearing to accept patients' own proposals and suggestions. As with the studies discussed above, these patients were unhappy with their doctors. A few patients, however, reported much more positive responses from doctors who managed to present their problems within an acceptable, i.e. biomedical framework. For example, depression could be presented as the result of biochemical abnormality and imbalance, rather than personal failure or incompetence. The ability of some doctors to connect with patients' search for a satisfactory interpretation of their distress was experienced as strongly positive and empowering.

Salmon, Peters & Stanley (1999) suggest that this kind of medical endorsement of the explanatory models preferred by patients is a justifiable strategy and merits widespread adoption. Increasing patient wellbeing and satisfaction with healthcare is an intrinsically worthwhile objective, and should also deliver the additional benefit of reducing the considerable demands which MUS patients make on healthcare resources. However, from the perspective of Wileman, May & Chew-Graham's GP respondents, such support would merely extend their already unwilling collusion with patients and a situation which they perceive to undermine their professional authority and judgement. Part of their problem, also, is that in appearing to legitimate an inappropriate biomedical diagnosis they are set on a path which is likely to extend an inappropriate use of resources, including diagnostic tests, specialist referrals and unwarranted treatment.

Punamaki and Kokko (1995a) found that the extent of agreement between doctor and patient regarding the diagnosis of illness was the best predictor of patients' satisfaction with the consultation. Tuckett *et al.*'s research (1985) supports this finding, and also established that there is often a convergence in the understanding of laymen and professionals, especially in dealing with relatively routine or familiar conditions. Patients were found to contribute to the success of many consultations by correctly anticipating what was wrong, and what needed to be done about it. This enabled them to fill in many of the gaps in their doctor's communication about diagnosis and treatment. Where they were not able to do this, however, or where they disagreed with their doctor's formulation of the problem, the consultation failed. Because they have been socialised into reproducing the role of conventionally passive patient, it is very difficult for participants to engage in open disclosure and communication in medical consultations. Patient taciturnity inhibits the development of professional reflexivity to patient perspectives and preferences (Donovan & Blake 2000). Where professionals remain unaware of the existence and importance of patient concerns, and the nature of the explanatory schemes which underlie them, it is not surprising that they do not attempt to elicit these in the consultation. Even where such attempts are made, it is likely that the constraints of the bureaucratic format will inhibit patients' responses, because of the anticipated risk of ridicule or censure, or simply because such a response is not perceived to be appropriate (Guadagnoli & Ward 1998; Pollock 2001; Punamaki & Kokko 1995a).

The reality of general practice is that many patients consult with vague, indeterminate and intractable symptoms and chronic conditions which can be hard to manage satisfactorily from the clinical perspective (Kleinman 1980; Kleinman 1986; May *et al*. 2004; Wileman, May & Chew-Graham 2002; Woivalin *et al*. 2004). Doctors tend to regard such cases as difficult (heartsink), and patients as manipulative and inadequate. Patients, on the other hand, struggle for legitimacy and for understanding. However, where patients and doctors are operating with different, perhaps even fundamentally incommensurable, explanatory models of illness, even a shared understanding is unlikely to resolve the problem (May *et al*. 2004). Improved communication and extended information are not in themselves sufficient to change the commitment of either side, given the implications involved for personal face and self-esteem. In this kind of situation, the issue for concordance is not so much about patients and doctors reaching an agreement about choice of treatment, but rather how conflicts over appropriate diagnosis and underlying explanatory schemas may be resolved.

The bureaucratic format seeks to protect face by containing conflict and disagreement. Participants seem to agree by not expressing anything to the contrary. Many medical encounters may be judged *successful* to the extent that they fulfil the participants' expectations, even if they fail to optimise health outcomes. Where people are inwardly unhappy, the outward masking of discontent enables face to be saved and relationships to be preserved, albeit uneasily. A problem with concordance is that it places additional demands on already difficult interactions, in explicitly raising differences and conflicting perspectives which may not easily be reconciled. It is not clear what the consequences of such continuing and *open* differences of opinion would be for the doctor–patient relationship.

Tuckett *et al*.'s study (1985) found that patients who were assertive in the consultation pursued a risky strategy. Those who asked questions and openly expressed their doubts succeeded in getting more information from their doctors, but at the cost of generating tension and conflict in the consultation which, as we have seen, the conventional interactive order is designed to avoid. In a rare study of applied concordance, Dowell, Jones and Snadden (2002) explored attitudes and medicines use with patients with known difficulties in adhering to treatment. They identified a zone of discomfort marking the transition between a diagnostic and a therapeutic encounter, when differences between the doctor and patient became exposed. However, they found that 14 of their 22 respondents achieved better clinical control or improved medicines use at a three month follow-up. The key issue for patients centred on illness acceptance rather than medicines use, and Dowell, Jones and Snadden suggested that an improvement in the doctor–patient relationship was a critical part of the improved outcome. They concluded that the increased investment in time and skills – for both patients and doctors – required for concordant consultations was justified in terms of both increased patient satisfaction and clinical benefit. However, it is not yet clear how realistic the wider application of concordance may be, especially for routine medical encounters.

From the perspective of concordance it is clear that interactive barriers are built into the organisation of communication and the structure of the consultation. The fear of losing face, the resort to negative politeness and the inhibition on empathy that this entails lead to the use of interactive strategies including avoidance, inference and silence. Patients and professionals collaborate in this process of containment. Participants in medical consultations are socialised to conform to strongly engrained norms of behaviour which inhibit the full and open disclosure of information and concerns, and the achievement of shared understandings about preferred actions and outcomes. Consequently, although the consultation may succeed as a social encounter, it often does not realise its therapeutic potential. The persistence of the bureaucratic format – even in the face of prolonged and active pressure for change – can be partly explained in terms of its success in enabling participants to overcome the difficulties of interaction which are intrinsic to medical consultations. Concordance requires doctors and patients to confront these difficulties, and thus goes against the grain of current etiquette and deeply engrained norms of interaction. To succeed as a strategy, concordance must be able to deliver clear and demonstrable benefits. It is against this background of inertia and resistance that we turn to consider the impact and potential of shared decision making between professionals and patients.

References

Asscher AW, Parr GD and Whitmarsh VB (1995) Towards the safer use of medicines. *BMJ.* **311**(14 October): 1003–5.

Barry C, Bradley C, Britten N, Stevenson F and Barber N (2000) Patients' unvoiced agendas in general practice consultations. *BMJ.* **320**: 1246–50.

Barry MJ, Mulley AG, Fowler FJ and Wennberg JW (1988) Watchful waiting vs immediate transurethral resection for symptomatic prostatism. *Journal of the American Medical Association.* **259**: 3010–17.

Bastian H (2003) Just how demanding can we get before we blow it? *BMJ.* **326**(14 June): 1277–8.

Beckman HB and Frankel RM (1984) The effect of physician behavior on the collection of data. *Annals of Internal Medicine.* **101**: 692–6.

Bellon JA and Fernandez-Asensio ME (2002) Emotional profile of physicians who interview frequent attenders. *Patient Education and Counselling.* **48**: 33–41.

Bloor MJ and Horobin GW (1975) Conflict and conflict resolution in doctor/patient interactions. In: C Cox and A Mead (eds) *A Sociology of Medical Practice.* Collier-MacMillan, London, pp. 271–84.

Bradley C (1992a) Factors which influence the decision whether or not to prescribe: the dilemma facing general practitioners. *British Journal of General Practice.* **42**: 454–8.

Bradley C (1992b) Uncomfortable prescribing decisions: a critical incident study. *BMJ.* **304**(1 February): 294–6.

Britten N (1994) Patient demand for prescriptions: a view from the other side. *Family Practice.* **11**(1): 62–6.

Britten N (1995) Patients' demands for prescriptions in primary care. *BMJ.* **310**(29 April): 1084–5.

Britten N (2004) Patients' expectations of consultations. *BMJ.* **328**(21 February): 416–17.

Britten N, Stevenson F, Barry C, Barber N and Bradley C (2000) Misunderstanding in prescribing decisions in general practice: a qualitative study. *BMJ.* **320**: 484–8.

Brown C, Dunbar-Jacob J, Palenchar DR, Kelleher KJ, Bruehlman RD, Sereika S and Thase ME (2001) Primary care patients' personal illness models for depression: a preliminary investigation. *Family Practice.* **18**(3): 314–20.

Brown P and Levinson S (1978) Universals in language usage: Politeness phenomena. In: EN Goody (ed.) *Questions and Politeness: strategies in social interaction.* Cambridge University Press, Cambridge, pp. 56–289.

Butler C, Rollnick S, Pill R, Maggs-Rapport F and Stott N (1998) Understanding the culture of prescribing: qualitative study of general practitioners' and patients' perceptions of antibiotics for sore throats. *BMJ.* **317**: 637–42.

Butler CC and Evans M (1999) The 'heartsink' patient revisited. *British Journal of General Practice.* **49**: 230–3.

Butler NM, Campion PD and Cox AD (1992) Exploration of doctor and patient agendas in general practice consultations. *Social Science and Medicine.* **35**(9): 1145–55.

Byrne PS and Long BEL (1976) *Doctors Talking to Patients.* HMSO, London.

Campion P and Langdon M (2004) Achieving multiple topic shifts in primary care medical consultations: a conversation analysis study in UK general practice. *Sociology of Health and Illness.* **26**(1): 81–101.

Cape J (2001) How general practice patients with emotional problems presenting with somatic or psychological symptoms explain their improvement. *British Journal of General Practice.* **51**(470): 724–9.

Cape J and McCullough Y (1999) Patients' reasons for not presenting emotional problems in general practice consultations. *British Journal of General Practice.* **49**: 875–9.

Cartwright A and Anderson R (1981) *General Practice Revisited: a second study of patients and their doctors.* Tavistock, London.

Chew-Graham CA and May C (1999) Chronic low back pain in general practice: the challenge of the consultation. *Family Practice.* **16**(1): 46–9.

Chew-Graham CA, Mullin S, May C, Hedley S and Cole H (2002) Managing depression in primary care: another example of the inverse care law? *Family Practice.* **19**(6): 632–7.

Cockburn J and Pitt S (1997) Prescribing behaviour in general practice: patients' expectations and doctors' perceptions of patients' expectations. *BMJ.* **315**: 520–30.

Cohen H and Britten N (2003) Who decides about prostate cancer treatment? A qualitative study. *Family Practice.* **20**(6): 724–9.

Coleman T, Murphy E and Cheater F (2000) Factors influencing discussion of smoking between general practitioners and patients who smoke: a qualitative study. *British Journal of General Practice.* **50**: 207–10.

Cornford CS (1998) Why patients consult when they cough: a comparison of consulting and non-consulting patients. *British Journal of General Practice.* **48**: 1751–4.

Coulter A (1997) Partnerships with patients: the pros and cons of shared decision-making. *Journal of Health Services Research and Policy.* **2**: 112–21.

Coulter A (2002) *The Autonomous Patient: ending paternalism in medical care.* The Nuffield Trust, London.

Cox K, Stevenson F, Britten N and Dundar Y (2004) *A Systematic Review of Communication Between Patients and Health Care Professionals About Medicine-taking and Prescribing.* Medicines Partnership, London.

Coyle J (1999) Exploring the meaning of 'dissatisfaction' with health care: the importance of 'personal identity threat'. *Sociology of Health and Illness*. **21**: 95–124.

Cromarty I (1996) What do patients think about during their consultations? A qualitative study. *British Journal of General Practice*. **46**: 525–8.

Department of Health (1991) *The Patient's Charter*. Department of Health, London.

Department of Health (1996) *Patient Partnership: building a collaborative strategy*. Department of Health, National Health Service Executive, London.

Department of Health (1998a) *In the Public Interest: developing a strategy for public participation in the NHS*. Department of Health NHS Executive, London.

Department of Health (1998b) *Our Healthier Nation: a contract for health*. Department of Health NHS Executive, London.

Department of Health (1999) *Patient and Public Involvement in the New NHS*. Department of Health, London.

Department of Health (2000) *The NHS Plan: a plan for investment, a plan for reform*. Department of Health, London.

Department of Health (2001a) *Involving Patient and the Public in Healthcare: a discussion document*. Department of Health, London.

Department of Health (2001b) *The Expert Patient: a new approach to chronic disease management for the 21st century*. Department of Health, London.

Department of Health (2002) *Learning from Bristol: the DH response to the report of the public inquiry into children's heart surgery at the Bristol Royal Infirmary 1984–1995*. Department of Health, London.

Department of Health (2003) *Building on the Best: choice, responsiveness and equity in the NHS*. Department of Health, London.

Dieppe P, Bartlett C, Davey P, Doyal L and Ebrahim S (2004) Balancing benefits and harms: the example of non-steroidal anti-inflammatory drugs. *BMJ*. **329**(3 July): 31–4.

Dixon-Woods M and Critchley S (1999) Medical and lay views of irritable bowel syndrome. *Family Practice*. **17**(2): 108–13.

Donovan J (1995) Patient decision making, The missing ingredient in compliance research. *International Journal of Technology Assessment in Health Care*. **11**: 443–55.

Donovan J and Blake D (2000) Qualitative study of interpretation of reassurance among patients attending rheumatology clinics: just a touch of arthritis, doctor? *BMJ*. **320**: 541–4.

Dowell J, Jones A and Snadden D (2002) Exploring medication use to seek concordance with 'non-adherent' patients: a qualitative study. *British Journal of General Practice*. **52**: 24–32.

Dowrick C (1992) Why do the O'Sheas consult so often? An exploration of complex family illness behaviour. *Social Science and Medicine*. **34**(5): 491–7.

Dowrick C and Buchan I (1995) Twelve month outcome of depression in general practice: does detection or disclosure make a difference? *BMJ*. **311**(11 November): 1274–6.

Dowrick C, May C, Richardson M and Bundred P (1996) The biopsychosocial model of general practice: rhetoric or reality? *British Journal of General Practice*. **46**: 105–7.

Ehrich K (2003) Reconceptualizing 'inappropriateness': researching multiple moral positions in demand for primary healthcare. *Health*. **7**(1): 109–26.

Eisenberg L (1978) Disease and illness: distinctions between professional and popular ideas of sickness. *Culture Medicine and Psychiatry*. **1**: 9–21.

Elwyn G, Edwards A and Kinnersley P (1999) Shared decision-making in primary care: the neglected second half of the consultation. *British Journal of General Practice*. **49**: 477–82.

Frankel S, Ebrahim S and Davey Smith G (2000) The limits to demand for health care. *BMJ*. **321**: 40–5.

Freeman AC and Sweeney K (2001) Why general practitioners do not implement evidence: qualitative study. *BMJ*. **323**(10): November, p. 1100.

Freidson E (1975) Dilemmas in the doctor/patient relationship. In: C Cox and A Mead (eds) *A Sociology of Medical Practice*. Collier MacMillan, London, pp. 285–98.

Gask L, Rogers A, Oliver D, May C and Roland M (2003) Qualitative study of patients' perceptions of the quality of care for depression in general practice. *British Journal of General Practice*. **53**: 278–83.

Gerrard TJ and Riddell JD (1988) Difficult patients: black holes and secrets. *BMJ*. **297**(20 August): 532–3.

Goffman E (1972) On face-work, an analysis of ritual elements in social interaction. In *Interaction Ritual, Essays on Face-to-Face Behaviour*. Penguin, Harmondsworth, pp. 5–45.

Goldberg D, Privett M, Ustan B, Simon G and Linden M (1998) The effects of detection and treatment on the outcome of major depression in primary care: a naturalistic study in 15 cities. *British Journal of General Practice*. **48**: 1840–4.

Groves JE (1978) Taking care of the hateful patient. *New England Journal of Medicine*. **298**(16): 883–7.

Guadagnoli E and Ward P (1998) Patient participation in decision-making. *Social Science and Medicine*. **47**: 329–39.

Hale AS (1997) Depression. *BMJ*. **315**: 43–6.

Henwood F, Wyatt S, Hart A and Smith J (2003) 'Ignorance is bliss sometimes': constraints on the emergence of the 'informed patient' in the changing landscapes of health information. *Sociology of Health and Illness*. **25**(6): 589–607.

Heritage J (1997) Conversation analysis and institutional talk, analysing data. In: D Silverman (ed.) *Qualitative Research, Theory, Method and Practice*. Sage, London, pp. 161–82.

Hirschfeld RM, Keller MB, Panico S, Arons BS, Barlow D, Davidoff F, Endicott J, Froom J *et al.* (1997) The National Depressive and Manic-Depressive Association consensus statement on the undertreatment of depression. *Journal of the American Medical Association*. **277**(4): 333–40.

Hunter MS and Britten N (1997) Decision making and hormone replacement therapy: a qualitative analysis. *Social Science and Medicine*. **45**: 1541–8.

Institute of Medicine (2000) *To Err is Human: building a safer health system*. National Academy Press, Washington DC. http://books.nap.edu/books/0309068371/html (accessed 28 September 2005).

Kadam UT, Croft P, McLeod J and Hutchinson M (2001) A qualitative study of patients' views on anxiety and depression. *British Journal of General Practice*. **51**: 375–80.

Kawachi I and Conrad P (1996) Medicalization and the pharmacological treatment of blood pressure. In: P Davis (ed.) *Contested Ground: public purpose and private interest in the regulation of prescription drugs*. Oxford University Press, Oxford, pp. 26–41.

Kettunen T, Poskiparta M, Liimatainen L, Sjogren A and Karhila P (2001) Taciturn patients in health counselling at a hospital: passive recipients or active participators? *Qualitative Health Research*. **11**(3): 399–410.

Kleinman A (1980) *Patients and Healers in the Context of Culture: an exploration of the borderland between anthropology, medicine and psychiatry*. University of California Press, Berkeley.

Kleinman A (1986) Concepts and a model for the comparison of medical systems as cultural systems. In: C Currer and M Stacey (eds) *Concepts of Health Illness and Disease: a comparative perspective*. Berg, Oxford.

Kleinman A (1988) *The Illness Narratives: suffering, healing and the human condition*. Basic Books, United States.

Korsch B and Negrete V (1972) Doctor patient communication. *Scientific American*. **227**(3): 66–74.

Kroenke K (2002) Psychological medicine. *BMJ*. **324**(29 June): 1536–7.

Lambert B (1995) Directness and deference in pharmacy students' messages to physicians. *Social Science and Medicine*. **40**(4): 545–55.

Ley P (1982) Satisfaction, compliance and communication. *British Journal of Clinical Psychology*. **21**: 241–54.

Ley P (1997) *Communicating With Patients: improving communication, satisfaction and compliance*. Stanley Thornes (Publishers) Ltd, Cheltenham.

Little P, Dorward M, Warner G, Stephens K, Senior J and Moore M (2004) Importance of patient pressure and perceived pressure and perceived medical need for investigations, referral, and prescribing in primary care: nested observational study. *BMJ*. **328**: 444.

Little P, Everitt H, Williamson I, Warner G, Moore M, Gould C, Ferrier K and Payne S (2001) Observational study of effect of patient centredness and positive approach on outcomes of general practice consultations. *BMJ*. **323**: 908–11.

Little P, Williamson I, Warner G, Gantley M and Kinmonth AL (1997) Open randomised trial of prescribing strategies in managing sore throat. *BMJ*. **314**: 722–7.

Makoul G, Arntson P and Schofield T (1995) Health promotion in primary care: physician–patient communication and decision making about prescription medications. *Social Science and Medicine*. **41**(9): 1241–54.

Marvel MK, Epstein RM, Flowers K and Beckman HB (1999) Soliciting the patient's agenda, have we improved? *Journal of the American Medical Association*. **281**(3): 283–7.

Maseide P (1991) Possibly abusive, often benign, and always necessary. On power and domination in medical practice. *Sociology of Health and Illness*. **13**(4): 545–61.

Mathers N, Jones N and Hannay D (1995) Heartsink patients: a study of their general practitioners. *British Journal of General Practice*. **45**: 293–6.

May C, Gayle A, Chapple A, Chew-Graham CA, Dixon C, Gask L, Graham R, Rogers A and Roland M (2004) Framing the doctor–patient relationship in chronic illness: a comparative study of general practitioner's accounts. *Sociology of Health and Illness*. **26**(2): 135–58.

Maynard DW (1991) Interaction and asymmetry in clinical discourse. *American Journal of Sociology*. **97**(2): 448–95.

McKevitt C and Morgan M (1997) Anomalous patients: the experiences of doctors with an illness. *Sociology of Health and Illness*. **19**(5): 644–67.

Medawar C (1997) The Antidepressant Web: marketing depression and making medicines work. *International Journal of Risk and Safety in Medicine*. **10**: 75–126.

Meredith P (1993) Patient satisfaction with communication in general surgery: problems of measurement and improvement. *Social Science and Medicine*. **37**(5): 591–602.

Montgomery SA *et al.* (1993) Guidelines for treating depressive illness with antidepressants. A statement from the British Association for Psychopharmacology. *Journal of Psychopharmacology*. **7**(1): 19–23.

Murray J and Corney R (1990) Not a medical problem? An intensive study of the attitudes and illness behaviour of low attenders with psychosocial difficulties. *Social Psychiatry and Psychiatric Epidemiology*. **25**: 159–64.

Neal RD, Heywood PL and Morley S (2000) 'I always seem to be there': a qualitative study of frequent attenders. *British Journal of General Practice*. **50**: 716–23.

O'Dowd TC (1988) Five years of heartsink patients in general practice. *BMJ*. **297**(20 August): 530–2.

Ohtaki S, Ohtaki T and Fetters MD (2003) Doctor–patient communication: a comparison of the USA and Japan. *Family Practice*. **20**(3): 276–82.

Pattenden J, Watt I, Lewin RJP and Stanford N (2002) Decision making processes in people with symptoms of acute myocardial infarction: qualitative study. *BMJ*. **324**(27 April): 1006.

Petit-Zeman S, Sandamas G and Hogman G (2001) *Doesn't It Make You Sick? Side effects of medicine and physical health concerns of people with severe mental illness*. London, NSF.

Pilnick A (1998) 'Why didn't you say just that?' Dealing with issues of asymmetry, knowledge and competence in the pharmacist/client encounter. *Sociology of Health and Illness*. **20**(1): 29–51.

Pirmohamed M, James S, Meakin S, Green C, Scott AK, Walley TJ, Farrar K, Park BK and Breckenridge AM (2004) Adverse drug reactions as cause of admission to hospital: prospective analysis of 18 820 patients. *BMJ*. **329**(3 July): 15–19.

Pollock K (2001) 'I've not asked him, you see, and he's not said': understanding lay explanatory models of illness is a prerequisite for concordant consultations. *International Journal of Pharmacy Practice*. 9(2): 105–18.

Pollock K and Grime J (2002) Patients' perceptions of entitlement to time in general practice consultations for depression: qualitative study. *BMJ*. 325(28 September): 687.

Prior L, Wood F, Lewis G and Pill R (2003) Stigma revisited, disclosure of emotional problems in primary care consultations in Wales. *Social Science and Medicine*. 56(10): 2191–200.

Punamaki, R-L and Kokko SJ (1995a) Content and predictors of consultation experiences among Finnish primary care patients. *Social Science and Medicine*. 40: 231–43.

Punamaki, R-L and Kokko SJ (1995b) Reasons for consultation and explanations of illness among Finnish primary-care patients. *Sociology of Health and Illness*. 17(1): 42–64.

Raine R, Carter S, Sensky T and Black N (2004) General practitioners' perceptions of chronic fatigue syndrome and beliefs about its management, compared with irritable bowel syndrome: qualitative study. *BMJ*. 328: 1354–7.

Rees Jones I, Berney L, Kelly M, Doyal L, Griffiths C, Feder G, Hillier S, Rowlands G and Curtis S (2004) Is patient involvement possible when decisions involve scarce resources? A qualitative study of decision-making in primary care. *Social Science and Medicine*. 59(1): 93-102.

Robins LS and Wolf FM (1988) Confrontation and politeness strategies in physician–patient interactions. *Social Science and Medicine*. 27(3): 217–21.

Robinson JD (2001) Closing medical encounters: two physician practices and their implications for the expression of patients' unstated concerns. *Social Science and Medicine*. 53: 639–56.

Rogers A, Hassell K and Nikolaas G (1999) *Demanding Patients? Analysing the use of primary care*. Open University Press, Buckingham.

Rogers A, May C and Oliver D (2001) Experiencing depression, experiencing the depressed: The separate worlds of patient and doctors. *Journal of Mental Health*. 10(3): 317–33.

Roter DL (2000) The medical visit context of treatment decision-making and the therapeutic relationship. *Health Expectations*. 3: 17–25.

Roter DL, Stewart M, Putnam SM, Lipkin M, Stiles W and Inui TS (1997) Communication patterns of primary care physicians. *Journal of the American Medical Association*. 277(4): 350–6.

Rycroft-Malone J, Latter S, Yerrell P and Shaw D (2001) Consumerism in health care: the case of medication information. *Journal of Nursing Management*. 9: 221–30.

Salmon P, Peters S and Stanley I (1999) Patients' perceptions of medical explanations for somatisation disorders: qualitative analysis. *BMJ*. 318(6 February): 372–6.

Schwartz RK, Soumeris B and Ajorn J (1989) Physician motivations for non-scientific drug prescribing. *Social Science and Medicine*. 28(6): 577–82.

Silverman D (1987) *Communication and Medical Practice*. Sage Publications, London.

Starland B (2001) New paradigms for quality in primary care. *British Journal of General Practice*. 51: 303–9.

Stevenson F, Barry C, Britten N, Barber N and Bradley C (2000) Doctor–patient communication about drugs: the evidence for shared decision making. *Social Science and Medicine*. 50: 829–40.

Stimson G (1974) Obeying doctor's orders: a view from the other side. *Social Science and Medicine*. 8: 97–104.

Stimson G and Webb B (1975) *Going to See the Doctor: the consultation process in general practice*. Routledge and Kegan Paul, London.

Stokes T, Dixon-Woods M and McKinley RK (2003) Breaking up is never easy: GPs' accounts of removing patients from their lists. *Family Practice*. 20(6): 628–34.

Stokes T, Dixon-Woods M and McKinley RK (2004) Ending the doctor–patient relationship in general practice: a proposed model. *Family Practice.* **21**(5): 507–14.

Strong P (1979) *The Ceremonial Order of the Clinic: patients, doctors and medical bureaucracies.* Routledge and Kegan Paul, London.

Tate P (2003) *The Doctor's Communication Handbook* (4e). Radcliffe Medical Press, Oxford.

Taylor C and White S (2000) *Practising Reflexivity in Health and Welfare: making knowledge.* Open University Press, Buckingham.

ten Have P (1991) Talk and social structure. In: D Boden and DH Zimmerman (eds) *Talk and Social Structure: studies in ethnomethodology and conversation analysis.* Polity Press, Cambridge, pp. 139–63.

Thompson A, Wilkinson G, Angst J, Kind P and Wade A (1996) Effective management of depression today: report from an interactive workshop. *International Journal of Clinical Psychopharmacology.* **11**(suppl 1): 45–50.

Tomlin Z, Humphrey C and Rogers S (1999) General practitioners' perceptions of effective health care. *BMJ.* **318**: 1532–5.

Tuckett D, Boulton M, Olson C and Williams A (1985) *Meetings Between Experts: an approach to sharing ideas in medical consultations.* Tavistock, London.

Tylee A (1995) How to improve depression detection rates. *Primary Care Psychiatry.* **1**: 9–13.

UMDS MSc in General Practice Teaching Group (1999) 'You're depressed'; 'No I'm not': GPs' and patients' different models of depression. *British Journal of General Practice.* **49**: 123–4.

Veldhuis M, Wigersma L and Okkes I (1998) Deliberate departures from good general practice: a study of motives among Dutch general practitioners. *British Journal of General Practice.* **48**: 1833–6.

Weiss M and Fitzpatrick R (1997) Challenges to medicine: the case of prescribing. *Sociology of Health and Illness.* **19**(3): 297–327.

Weiss M, Fitzpatrick R, Scott DK and Goldacre MJ (1996) Pressure on the general practitioner and decisions to prescribe. *Family Practice.* **13**(5): 432–8.

Weiss M and Scott D (1997) Whose rationality? A qualitative analysis of general practitioners' prescribing. *Pharmaceutical Journal.* **259**: 339–41.

Wennberg JE, Barry MJ, Fowler FJ and Mulley A (1993) Outcomes research, PORTs and health care reform. *Annals New York Academy of Sciences.* **703**: 52–62.

Werner A and Malterud K (2003) It is hard work behaving as a credible patient: encounters between women with chronic pain and their doctors. *Social Science and Medicine.* **57**: 1409–19.

Werner A, Widding Isaksen L and Malterud K (2004) 'I am not the kind of woman who complains of everything': Illness stories on self and shame in women with chronic pain. *Social Science and Medicine.* **59**: 1035–45.

Wileman L, May C and Chew-Graham CA (2002) Medically unexplained symptoms and the problem of power in the primary care consultation: a qualitative study. *Family Practice.* **19**(2): 178–82.

Wiles R and Higgins J (1996) Doctor–patient relationships in the private sector: patients' perceptions. *Sociology of Health and Illness.* **18**(3): 341–56.

Woivalin T, Krantz G, Mantyranta T and Ringsberg KC (2004) Medically unexplained symptoms: perceptions of physicians in primary health care. *Family Practice.* **21**(2): 199–203.

Zola IK (1981) Structural constraints in the doctor–patient relationship: the case of non-compliance. In: L Eisenberg and A Kleinman (eds) *The Relevance of Social Science for Medicine.* Reidel Publishing Company, Dordrecht, pp. 241–52.

Chapter Seven

Patient participation and shared decision making in the consultation

Patient–professional partnership and patient-centred care have become central to government health policy and regarded as a means to the delivery of better quality and more appropriate and cost-effective healthcare (Department of Health 1991, 1996, 1998, 1999, 2000, 2001a, 2001b; Hogg 1999). They reflect the emphasis on personal autonomy and institutional accountability in the modern state. The paternalism which has characterised professional delivery of healthcare from the inception of the National Health Service appears increasingly inappropriate and out of tune with the spirit of the times (Towle & Godolphin 1999). Traditional justifications for the professional to assume the role of 'perfect agent' (Gafni, Charles & Whelan 1998) of the patient in taking control of decisions about treatment and illness management have been substantially eroded. The monopoly of expert knowledge, the variability of clinical practice, the proliferation of therapeutic options, and uncertainty about their comparative efficacy and safety have undermined the social status of medical authority (Coulter 1997; Coulter 2002; Harrison & New 2002; Williams & Calnan 1996a; Williams & Calnan 1996b) (see Chapter 3). Given the risks and uncertainties involved, it is perceived to be unethical to exclude patients from choices which fundamentally affect their wellbeing and can only be determined in the context of individual values and preferences (Chewning & Wiederholt 2003; Hogg 1999; Wennberg et al. 1993).

Patient-centred medicine involves a shift in emphasis from the mechanics of treatment to the processes of care. It has been defined as:

> . . . the use of active listening skills by professionals; encouraging patients to express their agendas; attempting to understand patients' points of view and expectations; and working with patients in the management of their illness. Improving communication, meeting patients' information needs and sharing decisions can be seen as components of patient centred care.
>
> NHSCRD (2000: 2)

Patients' experience of care and *subjective* satisfaction with healthcare outcomes become important criteria for quality evaluation. This is deeply challenging to the traditional culture of medical paternalism. It calls for not just the acquisition of new (technical) skills in communication but also a major shift in perspective and vision, and this is much harder to realise.

The model of shared decision making (SDM) developed from the late 1990s as a means of conceptualising and promoting patient-centred practice (Charles, Gafni

& Whelan 1997; Charles, Whelan & Gafni 1999; Gafni, Charles & Whelan 1998). Charles *et al.* differentiated three basic forms of decision making in medical consultations. Paternalism is the traditional and still most characteristic type, in which the patient defers to medical expertise and judgement. Informed choice lies at the other end of the spectrum. The physician's task is to ensure that the patient is fully informed about his options, and thus in a position to make his own confident decisions about treatment. Shared decision making sits in between, involving both participants in a process of discussion, information sharing, negotiation and agreement about the best and most appropriate treatment to be adopted. Shared decision making is not necessarily the best option for medical encounters. Context and individual patient preferences will determine the most appropriate type of interaction and outcome. A single consultation may contain elements of more than one type of decision. The patient may willingly delegate decisions about treatment to his doctor in situations where he feels unable or unwilling to become involved himself. However, the model serves to make explicit the desirability of accommodating greater patient involvement, and points to the skills which both patient and professional need to learn and deploy in order to achieve this.

Good communication is critical for both patients and professionals to feel comfortable in exchanging views, negotiating decisions and, critically, to be reflexively aware of the other party's position and preferences. In this emphasis on shared understanding and negotiating decisions, the SDM and concordance models are very close to each other, and mutually reinforcing (Dowell 2004; Weiss 2004). Reflecting the particular interests of the working party responsible for originating the concept, and its subsequent association with the professionalisation project of pharmacy, concordance has been taken to apply particularly to decisions about the prescribing and use of medicines (RPSGB 1997). However, dividing up different stages and types of task and decision in the consultation in this way is unnecessarily restrictive and artificial. Limiting the applicability of concordance to medicines merely marginalises its relevance, rather than conferring a distinctive identity. The choice might refer to no treatment, or drugs as one among several possible options. It is consultations and relationships that are concordant, not just discussion or decisions about medicines. From this more inclusive perspective, the distinctive conceptual contribution of concordance is the acceptance that participants may have – and retain – contrasting positions and preferences that cannot be reconciled. Concordance recognises the existence of conflict in the consultation, and provides a means of dealing with it. The goal of a concordant consultation is not necessarily agreement, but rather recognition and understanding of each participant's point of view. Concordance goes further than the other models of decision making and patient participation in *acknowledging the reality* of patient primacy in decision making.

Shared decision making between patients and professional has come to be viewed as the fullest realisation of patient-centred care and the natural end point of active patient participation in the consultation. Advocates of shared decision making regard it as a satisfactory means of bringing together increased consumer involvement in healthcare, evidence-based decision making and egalitarian models of relationships between doctors and patients (Coulter 2002; Elwyn, Edwards & Kinnersley 1999; Guadagnoli & Ward 1998; Hope 1996).

Systematic lists of the skills or 'competences' required for professionals and patients to engage in shared decision making have been devised (Elwyn *et al.* 2000; Towle & Godolphin 1999). Although derived from consultation with lay and professional stakeholders, Towle and Godolphin's catalogue enumerates a formidable array of complex tasks and skills required of both patients and professionals (Box 7.1). Such formulas may have some value as aspirational statements for the development and evaluation of increased partnership in medical consultations. However, they are far removed from the contingencies and situational constraints governing real world encounters between doctors and patients. In particular, the interaction rules underpinning the dynamics of professional dominance and the structured asymmetry of the consultation which were reviewed in Chapter 6 highlight the great distance that remains to be closed between the current reality of most medical practice and the ideals of patient-centred medicine and concordance. Notwithstanding problems of recognition and evaluation, it is not surprising to find that there is widespread agreement that involvement of patients as active participants and decision makers in consultations remains uncommon.

Box 7.1 Physician and patient competencies for informed shared decision making

Physician
1 Develop a partnership with the patient.
2 Establish or review the patient's preferences for information (such as amount or format).
3 Establish or review the patient's preferences for role in decision making (such as risk taking and degree of involvement of self and others) and the existence and nature of any uncertainty about the course of action to take.
4 Ascertain and respond to patient's ideas, concerns, and expectations (such as about disease management options).
5 Identify choices (including ideas and information that the patient may have) and evaluate the research evidence in relation to the individual patient.
6 Present (or direct patient to) evidence, taking into account competencies 2 and 3, framing effects (how presentation of the information may influence decision making), etc. Help patient to reflect on and assess the impact of alternative decisions with regard to his values and lifestyle.
7 Make or negotiate a decision in partnership with the patient and resolve conflict.
8 Agree an action plan and complete arrangements for follow up.

Patients
1 Define (for oneself) the preferred doctor–patient relationship.
2 Find a physician and establish, develop and adapt a partnership.
3 Articulate (for oneself) health problems, feelings, beliefs, and expectations in an objective and systematic manner.
4 Communicate with the physician in order to understand and share relevant information (such as from competency 3) clearly and at the appropriate time in the medical interview.

5 Access information.
6 Evaluate information.
7 Negotiate decisions, give feedback, resolve conflict, agree on an action
   plan.

Towle and Godolphin (1999)*

A substantial body of research has confirmed that it is still rare for patients to play an active role in medical encounters and that most are reluctant to put forward an explicit statement of their preferences. Professionals seldom elicit patients' expectations or agendas in the consultation (Barry *et al.* 2000; Braddock *et al.* 1999; Britten *et al.* 2000; Butler *et al.* 1998; Cape & McCullough 1999; Cox *et al.* 2004; Elwyn, Edwards & Kinnersley 1999; Kettunen *et al.* 2001; Marvel *et al.* 1999; McKinley & Middleton 1999; Punamaki & Kokko 1995; Roter *et al.* 1997; Roter 2000; Stevenson *et al.* 2000). For example: Coulter *et al.* carried out a study of 425 women consulting their GPs about menorrhagia. They found that the doctors remained unaware of patients' preferences about treatment in 45% of cases. Even women who indicated that they had a clear choice of treatment were often unsuccessful in communicating these views to their doctor (Coulter, Peto & Doll 1994). Roter *et al.* found that two thirds of the 537 consultations they reviewed were physician-dominated and narrowly focused on medical, rather than patient, concerns (Roter *et al.* 1997). In another study, Braddock *et al.* found that only 9% of 3552 clinical decisions occurring in 1057 consultations met their criteria for fully informed patient decision making. More complex decisions were relatively uncommon, but were also the least likely to be informed. Patients were often told about the treatment or intervention to be imposed, but discussion of the reason for its selection, alternatives, or associated risks, benefits and uncertainties was unusual. Even where patients' preferences were elicited in the consultation, their understanding of the treatment decision was rarely checked or explored (Braddock *et al.* 1999). In the absence of clear discussion, it is apparent that professionals often make incorrect assumptions about what their patients want and expect from the consultation, and unilateral decisions about the best course of treatment (Altiner *et al.* 2004; Britten *et al.* 2000; Britten 2004; Butler, Campion & Cox 1992; Cockburn & Pitt 1997; Little *et al.* 2004; Wennberg *et al.* 1993).

Although the commitment to patient-centred medical practice can be justified on purely ethical and humanistic grounds, there is obviously interest in the extent to which this approach can deliver more concrete benefits (Elwyn *et al.* 2000; Guadagnoli & Ward 1998; Kaplan, Greenfield & Ware 1989; Towle & Godolphin 1999). Patients who are actively involved in discussion about treatment are assumed to be more committed to resulting decisions and so more likely to achieve better self-care, higher rates of adherence and consequent improvements in symptoms and physiological function. It seems intuitively reasonable that this should be the case, although it has proved difficult to establish this consistently, or to discover which aspects of patient-centred medical encounters may be responsible for producing concrete benefits. A number of frequently cited studies have found a connection between patient-centred consultations and

* Towle and Godolphin (1999) *BMJ.* **319**(18 September): 767, 768. Amended with permission from the BMJ Publishing Group.

improvements in physiological function or illness outcome (Cox *et al*. 2004; Fitzpatrick, Hopkins & Harvard-Watt 1983; Greenfield *et al*. 1988; Kaplan, Greenfield & Ware 1989; Little *et al*. 1999; Little *et al*. 2001; Rosenberg 1976; Stewart 1995). Greenfield, Kaplan and colleagues carried out a series of random controlled trials involving chronic patients suffering from diabetes, ulcer and hypertension. All three of these were consistent in finding that a training programme was effective in enabling patients to play a more active role in the consultation and communicate more effectively with their doctors. The intervention patients subsequently experienced better blood sugar/blood pressure control and reduced functional limitations compared to controls (Greenfield *et al*. 1988; Kaplan, Greenfield & Ware 1989). In a review of the literature, Stewart found a positive relationship between the quality of communication and a range of healthcare outcomes in 16 of 21 studies. These included emotional health, symptom resolution, physiological measures and pain control (Stewart 1995). Dowell *et al*. also reported a positive effect of enhanced communication between doctors and patients. They investigated the effects of extended consultations to discuss medicines use with 22 patients who had an established history of poor clinical control and 'suboptimal' medicines use. Fourteen of these were assessed as having improved clinical control or medicines use at three month follow-up (Dowell, Jones & Snadden 2002).

These studies point to at least the potential impact of the medical consultation, specifically the quality of the communication and relationship between patients and professionals, as a therapeutic intervention in its own right. It is difficult to identify or evaluate the contribution and importance of different aspects of patient-centredness, or precisely what it is that constitutes a 'good' relationship. For example, it may be that doctors who involve their patients in decisions are naturally better communicators, and it is this aspect of their behaviour, rather than the patient's assuming some responsibility for decision making, that is responsible for improving satisfaction and health outcome. The lack of definitional clarity and terminological precision, along with the methodological diversity of studies in this area, and the range and complexity of clinical situations to be evaluated, make it particularly difficult to compare results or establish consistent findings (Guadagnoli & Ward 1998; Mead & Bower 2002). To date, however, commitment to the benefits of patient-centred medicine and shared decision making seems to be running ahead of evidence of tangible benefit (Dowell 2004; Elwyn *et al*. 2000; Entwistle *et al*. 1998; Ford, Schofield & Hope 2002; Guadagnoli & Ward 1998). In an otherwise strongly evidence-based biomedical culture, the willingness to *anticipate* such findings in advance of delivery indicates the extent to which shared decision making and patient-centred medicine are supported by ideological and policy commitment rather than evidence.

Regardless of the desirability of patient-centred medicine, and assuming that it *can* deliver genuine benefits regarding both process and outcome of healthcare, many obstacles stand in the way of its general implementation. Patient-centred medicine, and shared decision making in particular, constitute a major challenge to professional practice (Dowell, Jones & Snadden 2002; Elwyn *et al*. 1999a; Elwyn *et al*. 2000). Several studies have indicated that both patients and doctors can learn to modify their behaviour in the consulting room (Dowell, Jones & Snadden 2002; Elwyn *et al*. 2004; Greenfield *et al*. 1988; Kaplan, Greenfield & Ware 1989). However, the evidence also suggests that patient activity is associated with an increased likelihood of tension and conflict, rather than heightened satisfaction. Patient participation may thus be recognised as a risky strategy, and best avoided as a means of protecting participants' mutual investment in their long-term relationship. The discussion of structured asymmetry and the negotiated order of medical consultations in Chapter 6 has pointed to the strongly entrenched situational and interactional constraints on cultural and behavioural change of both patients and doctors. To the extent that a patient-centred perspective has made inroads into practice, it seems to have been largely confined to tasks which Elwyn *et al.* have characterised as belonging to the 'first half' of the consultation: establishing empathy with patients and formulating the problem. The patient is rarely involved in the neglected 'second half', in which management options are identified and decisions about treatment are made (Elwyn, Edwards & Kinnersley 1999). Neither participants are accustomed to patients sharing decisions about treatment. Patients often have difficulty in accepting a more active role in the consultation, while professionals are unwilling to accept that patients have sufficient competence to make complex judgements about treatment.

The interactional dominance enjoyed by professionals clearly gives them the edge in neutralising or even subverting the patient-centredness of consultations. Doctors can often rely on patient taciturnity and deference and thus appear to offer choice and involvement which patients are unprepared for, and consequently fail to take up. This strategy of 'pseudoconcordance' is a recognised means of manipulating patients. For example, questions such as 'What would you like me to do for you' may function as rhetorical devices rather than genuine enquiries. This is a difficult, if not impossible, question for patients to answer, in view of the felt inappropriateness of expressing such ideas and suggestions to 'experts'. It constitutes a face-threatening act and nicely exposes the patient double bind, i.e. the requirement to exercise good judgement about when it is necessary to seek medical attention, but suspend it thereafter (Bloor & Horobin 1975). Thrown off guard, the patient can only reply with some version of 'I don't know (you're the doctor)' – at least if he is to stick to the rules. Having made an offer that the patient does not know how to take up, the doctor not only stifles any threat of further resistance but reinforces his professional authority, and is then free to pursue his own agenda (Elwyn *et al.* 1999a; Gwyn & Elwyn 1999). The interactional dominance of professionals in setting the limits of shared decision making is explored by Gwyn and Elwyn in analysis of a consultation involving a child suffering from an upper respiratory tract infection. The discourse between the patient's father and the doctor is framed in terms of patient choice. However, the father's preference (antibiotics for a throat infection that the doctor considers to be probably viral in origin, despite a declared diagnosis of 'tonsillitis') is not acceptable to the doctor. It is apparent throughout the consultation that the doctor is using the linguistic devices of interactional dominance to (successfully) pursue his covert agenda to persuade the parents to abandon their quest for antibiotics (Elwyn *et al.* 1999b; Gwyn & Elwyn 1999).

The strategy of constraining and directing patient choice through the selective presentation and 'framing' of information has been widely reported (Cox *et al.* 2004; Dowell 2004; Edwards, Elwyn & Mulley 2002; Elwyn *et al.* 1999a; Freeman & Sweeney 2001; Maynard 1991; Rees Jones *et al.* 2004; Silverman 1987a). Stapleton, Kirkham & Thomas' study of the influence of information leaflets on informed choice in maternity units also illustrates the extent to which factors relating to organisational and professional hierarchy may restrict patients' awareness and capacity to become involved in their care (Stapleton, Kirkham & Thomas 2002) (see also Pollock *et al.* 2004). The norms of clinical practice were defined by the (highest ranking) obstetricians, which resulted in mothers being channelled to accept technological interventions. Staff were selective about which leaflets were made accessible to patients. Junior staff felt unable to deviate from the standard practice of the clinic or oppose the authority of senior colleagues, and so would not support mothers who wanted to resist this. The end result was that patients collaborated with 'informed compliance' rather than 'informed choice' even though, in principle, staff supported their entitlement to make their own decisions about care. In other contexts it is evident that clinicians may be self-consciously aware of their deliberate manipulation of information as a way of securing patient compliance with professional decisions (Elwyn *et al.* 1999a; Freeman & Sweeney 2001; Rees Jones *et al.* 2004).

The phenomenon of framing highlights the greatest stumbling block to the widespread realisation of shared decision making: that professionals are only prepared to accept patient preferences when these correspond to clinically 'acceptable' decisions. From the prescriber's perspective it is deeply problematic to acquiesce in choices of treatment that are deemed to be 'bad', or inappropriate (Dowell 2004; Ford, Schofield & Hope 2002; Gwyn & Elwyn 1999). For example, in the case analysis of the child presenting with the throat infection, Gwyn and Elwyn support the doctor's manipulation of the consultation to achieve the clinically preferred outcome of not prescribing antibiotics: where the patient choice is 'incorrect' it is appropriate to depart from shared decision making. They go on to argue (somewhat perplexingly) that this disregard of the patient's preference for treatment actually 'enriches' the shared decision making process. The risk of patient choice is underwritten by medical judgement and expertise (Gwyn & Elwyn 1999). Patients are only allowed to make choices when these represent their own 'best interests' (as judged by professionals). Professional concern about the adverse physiological consequences of patients opting for 'bad' or inappropriate treatments and outcomes is expressed alongside the clinching override that choice should only be extended provided patients demonstrate a competence which it remains the professional prerogative to judge (Dowell 2004). In effect, patient preferences can be ruled out of many of the major areas in which treatment decisions are likely to be contentious from a clinical perspective. In this professional formulation, far from contributing to a more egalitarian relationship, shared decision making risks merely providing a shield for the continuation of a medical paternalism which is all the more insidious for being masked by the front of (illusory) patient choice and the semblance of involvement in the consultation.

Glyn and Elwyn propose that shared decision making is restricted in its application to areas of 'clinical equipoise' where (from the clinical standpoint) there are several viable and equally appropriate or effective treatment alternatives from which the patient may select according to personal preference (Elwyn *et al.* 1999b; Elwyn *et al.* 2000; Gwyn & Elwyn 1999). Clinical equipoise occurs, in other words, in situations where the clinician lacks either certainty or concern. These include the treatment of menorrhagia, atrial fibrillation, prostate disease and menopausal symptoms. Increasingly, also, patient choice is likely to be further restricted by the impact of national guidelines in suppressing doctors' presentation of dispreferred treatment options.

Evidently, it is hard even for professionals who are sympathetic to the principles of shared decision making and concordance to accept that patients can be competent to make sound decisions about their healthcare (Thorne, Ternulf Nyhlin & Paterson 2000). This lack of trust might be understandable if professionals themselves could be confidently assumed always to provide appropriate and effective care. However, as the discussion of medical error and inconsistency in Chapter 3 has made clear, this is very far from being the case. The resort to clinical judgement as the final arbiter in medical decision making exemplifies the disadvantage of professional dominance that shared decision making is intended to reduce. Where professionals are not challenged to deal with patient preferences which constitute 'uncomfortable prescribing incidents' they remain unaware of the nature and significance of the explanatory models and rationales underlying the patient perspective. As a result, they continue to operate with inaccurate and inappropriate stereotypes of patient wants and motives, and to orient medical practice towards a narrowly technical and instrumental form of rationality. Whilst there is widespread concern about unnecessary and inappropriate prescribing of antibiotics, the literature also indicates that some doctors judge this to be an appropriate response (i.e. a legitimate trade-off) in situations where the dictates of 'rational' prescribing are subordinated to the achievement of other goals such as patient satisfaction or protecting the long-term relationship with patients in order to secure acceptance of other, perhaps more important, decisions in future (Butler *et al.* 1998; Schwartz, Soumeris & Ajorn 1989; Tomlin, Humphrey & Rogers 1999; Veldhuis, Wigersma & Okkes 1998; Weiss & Scott 1997).

Professional concerns about patients' bad choices and inappropriate demand display a lack of awareness of the patient perspective. As was discussed earlier, there is considerable evidence that inappropriate prescribing of antibiotics derives substantially from the inaccurate assumptions which doctors often make about patient expectations of treatment, rather than their actual preferences. Patients are prescribed more antibiotics than they want or expect. In fact, far from avidly pursuing 'a pill for every ill', lay aversion to taking medicines, especially unnecessarily, is well established (Britten *et al.* 2004). The persistence of widespread non-compliance with prescribed treatment is a cogent testimony to the public's dislike of taking medicines, and their disagreement with their doctors' decisions about treatment.

Dowell (2004) states the crux of the prescriber's dilemma in relation to concordance: the difficulty for professionals in deferring to patient decisions and treatment use which violates what they regard to be 'best practice', especially when patients may suffer adverse outcomes as a result. However, we might ask: what is the point of professionals prescribing medicines which patients do not, or no longer want to, take? The outcome, in physiological terms, is likely to be the same. However, if patient preferences and intentions are made clear in a 'concordant' consultation, not only will unnecessary prescriptions be avoided, but the commitment to increased patient autonomy and self-determination will be honoured, and the relationship between patient and prescriber may well be strengthened as a result. In reality, patients do not often lightly disregard professional advice. The premise (and perhaps also the promise) of concordance is that strong relationships and shared understandings are more likely to result in patients acceding to their doctors' recommendations, rather than rejecting them. Patient compliance with medical advice may even be extended, rather than diminished, as a result. The point is that patient priorities and judgements about what is most important to maintaining quality of life do not necessarily accord with clinical best practice. Where there is a clash between these perspectives, concordance recognises the practical and ethical grounds for reversing traditional priorities, and privileging the patient, rather than the professional, perspective. This point is well illustrated in Reis *et al.*'s account of a case where the patient's rejection of her consultant's recommendation to take warfarin was negotiated through the written accounts of the feelings and responses which she and her family doctor shared with each other. This lady preferred to live independently of medication and to accept that she might increase her risk of having a stroke as a result.

> With every pill I put in my mouth, I feel I'm poisoning myself . . . I felt in the consultation with the cardiologist my feelings and wishes were not even considered. . . . You did say, however, that in the end it **is** my decision . . . I will have to take charge of and live my life with no pills for as long as I can . . . no chance that, if my situation stays the way it is now, I will take more or stronger medications [i.e. warfarin] . . .
>
> Reis *et al.* (2002: 1019)*

The doctor retained his professional misgivings, but accepted the patient's decision.

> Three family meetings were held during the course of one month. We shared information. We discussed our feelings. I respect that personal 'health belief model', which is definitely different from my own. She wants to be guided by her inner feelings rather than by fear, and she finally decides no to warfarin, yes to atenolol, and yes to aspirin. Fully aware of the possible risks in this course of action, her husband shares her decision. I feel I can live with it too.
>
> Reis *et al.* (2002: 1019)

Both, apparently, valued the strengthening of their relationship that such mutual understanding produced (Reis *et al.* 2002: 1019). Interestingly, the patient indicated her reflexive awareness and understanding of the anxieties her decision caused her doctor, and his sense of responsibility for providing good care. In the end, she opts for what she considers to be the lesser of two evils, in prioritising her sense of autonomy over dependence on toxic, albeit risk reducing, medication. It is evident, also, that she retains considerable regard for her doctor's opinion, and the door remains open for further discussion and possible revision of her decision in future. Her doctor reflects on the case:

> The patient's beliefs, preferences, and family members' input were much more powerful than the rational evidence. I took part in the process without a sense of professional compromise. The final appropriate decision for the specific dilemma with that particular patient can

* Reis S, Hermoni D, Livingstone P and Borkan J (2002) Case report of paroxysmal atrial fibrillation and anticoagulation. *BMJ*. **325**(2 November):1018–20. Reproduced with permission from the BMJ Publishing Group.

be contrary to the apparent evidence. Looking for evidence and sharing narratives served our relationship. Progress was made on the way to a more mindful practice.

Reis *et al.* (2002: 1019)

Lay commitment to the value of *enjoying life* and an awareness of the iatrogenic impact of medication in undermining the sense of wellbeing and personal autonomy required to do this, are important reasons for patients' resisting the medications their doctors prescribe for them. Even minor side effects from medication can have a substantial impact on patients' quality of life (Protheroe *et al.* 2000). Sachs describes the negative effect on wellbeing associated with awareness of raised cholesterol levels following routine screening in her sample of 40 year old Swedish farmers. The resulting fear and anxiety eroded individuals' confidence in their health and destroyed the trust they had in the physical integrity of their bodies. Enjoyment of life was further undermined by the effort to implement recommended lifestyle changes, which did not necessarily succeed in reducing cholesterol levels. Patient rejection of medical treatments and interventions is not, as professionals commonly suppose, the product of mindless ignorance or incapacity. Rather, it results from the application of a different kind of rationality, reflecting different priorities and values from those pursued in clinical medicine.

Bringing patient perspectives and preferences into the frame requires the reconsideration, and a widening, of what constitutes both 'best interests' and 'harm'. There is considerable evidence that, especially when adequately informed about the marginal gains and associated risks associated with many treatments, patients tend to be more conservative and risk-averse than their doctors (Coulter 2002; Deyo 2000; Edwards, Elwyn & Mulley 2002; Howitt & Armstrong 1999; Misselbrook & Armstrong 2001; Protheroe *et al.* 2000). Wennberg *et al.* (1993) found that patients' preferences in relation to treatment options for benign prostatic hyperplasia (BPH) were very variable, and bore no relation to the severity of symptoms experienced. When patients who had worked through an interactive computer program informing them about BPH and their treatment options (surgery, drugs or watchful waiting) were allowed to choose, they elected for a substantially lower rate of surgery than had formerly been practised by their surgeons. Patients clearly valued the risks associated with surgery (including impotence and incontinence) more negatively than the discomfort of continuing symptoms. The previously higher rate of surgery as well as the widespread variation in its incidence reflected the preferences ('best practice') of professionals, and contrasted with the patient choice of more conservative management of their condition (Barry *et al.* 1997; Wennberg *et al.* 1993). This imposition of professional preferences over patient choice in such circumstances is not only unwarranted but potentially harmful.

Far from giving rise to unrealistic expectations and unmanageable demand for healthcare, the evidence suggests that more active involvement of patients in decision making could reduce the amount of unnecessary or inappropriate drugs prescribed and taken. Instead of opening up the floodgates of unbridled demand, increasing patient involvement in healthcare decisions may actually reduce overall demand for services and associated costs, as well as increasing the quality of care (Coulter 1997; Coulter 2002; Frankel, Ebrahim & Davey Smith 2000;

O'Connor & Edwards 2001). In their review of the literature, O'Connor *et al.* found that, on average, well informed patients who were given the option were 26% less likely to accept major surgical intervention (O'Connor *et al.* 1999).

It is evident that patients are likely to make *different* choices from their doctors, especially when they are adequately informed about available alternatives. As we have seen, this can be very challenging to the professional perspective. The current conventions of the consultation and the professional dominance of the interaction facilitates the selective presentation and framing of information presented to patients. It is often only in the process of learning and reflection that patients develop their agenda and formulate their preferences. Evidence-Based Patient Choice has been advocated as a means of bridging the gap between evidence-based and patient-centred medicine. Decision aids have been developed as structured tools to help patients formulate their individual preferences and values in the light of the best currently available evidence about the benefits and harms of treatment (Deyo 2000; Edwards & Elwyn 2001; Ford, Schofield & Hope 2002; Hope 1996; O'Connor *et al.* 1999). Wennberg *et al.* (1993) were among the first to employ structured decision aids as a means of eliciting the treatment preferences for patients suffering from prostate disease (Box 7.2). As discussed above, their research revealed both the variability of patients' choice of treatment, and their greater caution and conservatism in relation to surgery: patient choice resulted in a significant reduction in the rate of operations performed.

Box 7.2 A shared decision making program for men facing a treatment decision for benign prostatic hyperplasia

Patients receive an introductory brochure and complete a short question-naire. Items of personal information including health status and symptoms are input into a computer to enable the program to be tailored to each individual. Patients watch a 30 minute presentation about available treat-ment options (watchful waiting, chemotherapy or surgery). Estimates of outcome probabilities are given both verbally and graphically. The next phase of the programme is a more interactive segment that allows patients to review earlier information and work through a series of optional modules dealing with acute retention, sexual dysfunction, incontinence, likely out-comes of surgery, the relationship between BPH and prostate cancer, blood transfusion and new treatments. A summary of the information reviewed is printed for the patient to take away, and a second copy is filed with his notes as a basis for shared knowledge and discussion between the patient and his doctor during subsequent consultations.

Source: Barry *et al.* 1997

The wider development and utilisation of information tools such as decision aids is welcomed as a means of ensuring that patients are presented with a range of risk portrayals rather than the more common or 'persuasive' ones (e.g. relative rather than absolute frequencies). Decision aids have the advantage that patients may use them independently as a resource outside the consultation, and take time to reflect and consider their position and/or as a prompt for discussion with their doctors. In addition to encouraging and structuring patient involvement in decision making, decision aids can also signal that it is *legitimate* for patients to possess information and so provide a pretext and opportunity for discussion with their doctors. A review of 17 RCTs involving decision aids concluded that they were effective in increasing patient knowledge and participation in decision making, without increasing anxiety (O'Connor *et al.* 1999). However, their effect on patients' satisfaction with their decision and the decision making process is less clear.

Bekker, Hewison & Thornton investigated the effect of decision aids on women who had screened positive for Down's syndrome and were then confronted with difficult decisions about whether or not to accept additional diagnostic tests and the further consequences of these (Bekker, Hewison & Thornton 2003). Their findings indicated that the decision aid was associated with more effective decision making and long-term decisional satisfaction. However, women found participating in the decision aid consultation challenging, and less satisfying compared with those who experienced routine care. Bekker, Hewison & Thornton conclude that such consultations are likely to be experienced as more difficult and less rewarding for both staff and patients, as they evoke greater immediate decisional conflict and negative emotion in the process of focused evaluation and choice.

Increased patient participation in the consultation and the redistribution of responsibility for decisions about healthcare can be a positive but also challenging experience for both patients and professionals. Elwyn and Charles (2001) observe that consultations featuring shared decision making contain a moment of expressed uncertainty by the doctor. This indication of equipoise offers the patient the opportunity to become involved in the discussion and choice of treatment. The expression of professional uncertainty may be face-threatening for the doctor and possibly perplexing and unwelcome to the patient (Edwards, Elwyn & Mulley 2002; Elwyn *et al.* 1999a; Holmes-Rovner *et al.* 2000). The practice of patient-centred medicine and shared decision making increases the complexity of the consultation, overturns the controlled conventions of the bureaucratic format and imposes additional demands on all participants. In their study of applied concordance, Dowell, Jones and Snadden commented on the tension generated by the exposure of the different and conflicting views held by patients and doctors. This 'zone of discomfort' marked the transition from a diagnostic to a therapeutic consultation (Dowell, Jones & Snadden 2002). Alongside the ingrained routines of the bureaucratic format, the added difficulties and complexities of concordant consultations constitute another reason for its limited take up among patients as well as professionals. Although the intrinsic desirability – perhaps even inevitability – of patient-centred medicine is widely assumed, little attention has been paid to how patients view and have responded to this initiative.

The traditional roles of patient and doctor may be restrictive, but they are relatively straightforward. Patient-centred medicine increases the complexity of consultations, and makes greater demands on all participants. Patient preferences for information and involvement may change over time and between different contexts of illness type, duration and severity (Patel, Mirsadraee & Emberton 2003; Paterson, Russell & Thorne 2001). Stated preferences may vary depending on whether people are well or ill when their opinion is sought. It is likely, also, that patients' responses will differ in primary and secondary care settings. Some types of health problems lend themselves to patient involvement more than others. Indeed, a spur to the development of patient-centred medicine has undoubtedly been the increase in numbers of people suffering from enduring chronic and degenerative illness. The day-to-day management of these conditions often requires a substantial input from the patient and perhaps also his carers. Patients are likely to become increasingly critical, assertive and involved in their care as they acquire experience and confidence in managing their illness and dealing with health service staff and agencies (Cohen & Britten 2003; Patel, Mirsadraee & Emberton 2003; Paterson, Russell & Thorne 2001; Silverman 1987b; West 1976).

Whilst it is a common finding that patient demand for information is increasing, the extent and frequency of patient desire to participate more actively in consultations is much less certain (Charles *et al.* 1998; Fallowfield 2001; Gafni, Charles & Whelan 1998; Kenny *et al.* 1999; Silverman 1987b; Strull, Lo & Charles 1984). It is not clear to what extent this reflects reflective choice or lack of awareness and familiarity with the skills and 'competencies' required for effective decision making (Coulter, Peto & Doll 1994; Kenny *et al.* 1999; Towle & Godolphin 1999). There is evidence that along a continuum of illness severity, patients are much more likely to prefer active involvement at the milder end. Those suffering from severe and life-threatening conditions often wish to delegate responsibility for treatment choice and management to professionals (Broadstock & Michie 2000; Burkitt Wright, Holcombe & Salmon 2004; Cohen & Britten 2003; de Haes & Koedoot 2003; Galletari, Butow & Tattersall 2001; Paterson, Russell & Thorne 2001; Silverman 1987b). However, patients may still feel the need to understand the rationale for clinical decisions, even if they prefer not to take part in these directly (Cohen & Britten 2003; Kenny *et al.* 1999). They might also confront the difficult task of negotiating the transition between more active and passive positions in response to fluctuations in their illness severity.

In some cases patients simply defer to professional expertise because they realise that they are out of their depth, and lack the competence to make judgements about highly complex and technical matters. Concern to behave appropriately as a 'good' patient and to avoid alienating staff is another reason for adopting a conventionally passive stance. The particular vulnerability of illness intensifies patient concern to retain the goodwill of their doctors (*see* Chapter 6). In addition, however, it is apparent that patients may have positive reasons for withdrawing from active involvement in decision making about treatment. Burkitt-Wright, Holcombe & Salmon describe the desire of breast cancer patients to relinquish responsibility and establish relationships of trust with their doctors, within which they could accept a dependent position as passive recipients of care. Some respondents regarded active involvement in decision making to be incompatible with trust in their doctors, which they felt to be a higher priority (Burkitt Wright, Holcombe & Salmon 2004). Radley describes the difficulties experienced by cardiac surgery patients in coming to terms with an operation which they perceived they had 'no option' but to accept. One of the ways patients coped with the threat of surgery was by investing their surgeons with a degree of skill and expertise. Trust in the competence of their doctors underpinned their confidence in the outcome of their operation (Radley 1996). Similarly, Salkeld *et al.* found that cancer patients' trust in the skill and competence of their surgeon was the most important factor underlying their confidence that the best treat-ment decision had been made. Their trust was founded on good and open communication and emotional support, rather than the provision of technical information about treatment (Salkeld *et al.* 2004).

The desire of patients to distance themselves from decisions which may have a momentous impact on their wellbeing has been noted in a number of other studies. By delegating the responsibility patients can to some extent protect themselves against regret and personal reproach if decisions subsequently turn out to be 'wrong' (Charles *et al.* 1998; Edwards, Evans & Elwyn 2003; Kenny *et al.* 1999; McPherson 1994; Patel, Mirsadraee & Emberton 2003; Salkeld *et al.* 2004; Silverman 1987b). The urge to surrender to professional authority has been noted among doctors whose experience of illnesses obliges them to adopt the role of patient (Ingelfinger 1980; McKevitt & Morgan 1997). Coyle found that for some patients relinquishing power in situations of great vulnerability and uncertainty could result in an *increased* sense of control. There was, however, a great difference between voluntarily giving up power and having it taken away. Patients were extremely critical of what they regarded as coercive and paterna-listic behaviour by their doctors. This was experienced as a major identity threat and profoundly disempowering, extreme enough to provoke formal complaint (Coyle 1999).

The movement towards patient-centred medicine and shared decision making has acquired the force of moral imperative (Coulter 2002; Makoul 1998; May & Mead 1998). The democratisation of outmoded medical paternalism is viewed as intrinsically desirable for ethical reasons, as well as promising to deliver better health outcomes. It has been assumed that retaining a sense of personal control is an important adaptive response to the experience of illness, and that actively involving patients in decision making about care will improve their experience of care and ability to cope with illness (Galletari, Butow & Tattersall 2001). However, doubts are being voiced about the extent to which such autonomy is necessarily beneficial, or actually in line much of the time with what patients actually want (Paterson, Russell & Thorne 2001; Salmon & Hall 2004). The studies considered above indicate that it is not so much active involvement and choice of treatment that patients are looking for in their dealings with health professionals, as empathetic acknowledgement and support.

The provision of information and discussion about management decisions and treatment choices may be valued for their part in building good relationships and demonstrating professional interest and respect for the patient as person, rather than for their role in promoting patient autonomy. What seems to matter most to patients is the feeling that they have been dealt with considerately, perhaps even the *sense* of involvement, rather than involvement itself; the illusion, rather than the exercise, of choice. For example, in a focus group study of patient preferences in healthcare, respondents indicated their desire to feel that they had been able to contribute meaningfully to a consultation in which their opinions and feelings had been taken into account. They felt it was important that they understood and agreed with the choice of treatment, but perceived involvement in decision making was more important than active engagement. These ideas express the importance to these respondents of feeling that they have been treated with respect and consideration by their doctors. Thus, while it might be unrealistic for patients to be presented with *all* relevant information, it was nevertheless important to feel that an option had been approved – with perhaps the theoretical possibility of rejection – rather than arbitrarily imposed (Edwards *et al.* 2001). Other studies have also reported the importance of respondents' sense of formally *having* an option, even if in practice, they routinely acquiesce in their doctor's choice of treatment (Burkitt Wright, Holcombe & Salmon 2004).

Within the context of a wide variation in patient preferences for information and active involvement in consultations it is evident that the assumption that shared decision making represents the most complete and desirable manifestation of patient-centred medicine needs to be revised. The research findings discussed above suggest that while patients may often want more open communication with their doctors, they are much more concerned with the *affective* aspects of their relationship than gaining control over the instrumental or technical aspects of treatment (Lupton 1997). It may be that patients experience empathy rather than autonomy to be the critical feature of healthcare. Rather than being always arbitrary and abusive, professional power is seen to be potentially benign and constructive, and traditional paternalism to confer some benefit to the patient (Lupton 1997; Maseide 1991). Quill and Brody advocate a goal of 'enhanced autonomy', which seems very close to the basic principles of concordance. This provides scope for patients' informed choice, but without aiming to deny the reality of the power disparity – both technical and interactive – between patients and doctors. Through an open disclosure of his preferences, the doctor may substantially neutralise the effect of his personal bias, while enabling the patient to benefit from professional skill and expertise.

> An open dialogue, in which the physician frankly admits his or her biases, is ultimately a better protector of the patient's right to autonomous choice than artificial neutrality would be.
>
> Quill & Brody (1996)*

As in concordance, patients and professionals may not change their preferences or decisions in the course of an 'enhanced autonomy discussion', but they may achieve a better understanding of each other's position (Quill & Brody 1996) as well as reappraising the meaning and significance of the decisions made.

Silverman proposes that the medical encounter *depends* on a differential of power between the doctor and patient. To challenge this destroys the role and purpose of the encounter: why should patients seek or follow advice from people who are not differentiated by their greater expertise and knowledge? In this view, reducing the structured asymmetry in the relationship between patient and professional risks destroying the form of the consultation and with it the benefit to be derived from traditional paternalism (Lupton 1997; Silverman 1987b). Lupton also supports the view that the drive to extend patient consumerism may work to patients' disadvantage if it destroys public confidence and faith in professional expertise. She describes the tension between patients' desire for autonomy and their need to relinquish control in a cultural context where self-reliance is valorised and dependency signifies weakness. When people are sick and weak and vulnerable autonomy is no longer a priority: they seek help.

---

* Quill TE and Brody H (1996) Physician recommendations and patient autonomy: finding a balance between physician power and patient choice. *Annals of Internal Medicine.* **125**(9): 763–9.

Dependency is intrinsic to the experience of illness. Patients' trust in their doctors and faith in medical expertise has always been an important component of the medical encounter. However, the modern patient is caught between the desire to maintain autonomy and the desire to evade responsibility – and consequently, also, moral accountability – for dealing with illness. Lupton concludes that in their dealings with health professionals, patients will tend to move between the opposing positions of active decision maker and passive subject according to context (Bishop & Yardley 2004; Lupton 1997).

Alongside the view that traditional paternalism confers some benefits for patients, the argument has emerged that the move to patient-centred medicine can actually intensify the disadvantage of some patients, in the course of furthering professional self-interest. Salmon and Hall (2003) suggest that the increasing transfer of responsibility for health management and treatment decisions to patients enables professionals to reduce their own involvement in care (*see also* Dowrick 1999). This contraction of accountability relates particularly to problematic areas of medical work which medicine can do little to alleviate, such as chronic disease and pain, mental illness and medically unexplained symptoms. Far from being empowered, patients are likely to find themselves implicated in the genesis of their own problems, struggling to establish their credibility as legitimate patients and handed the task of managing their recovery (Werner & Malterud 2003; Werner, Widding Isaksen & Malterud 2004). For example, Salmon and Hall (2004) describe patient responses to the use of post-operative patient controlled anaesthesia (PCA). This should be a good idea, because such pain relief is known to be often inadequate due to a combination of patients' reluctance to request it and nurses' inability to accurately assess the severity of patients' discomfort (Salmon & Manyande 1996). PCA is supposed to improve pain relief and 'empower' patients by providing push button control over the release of an intravenously administered opoid. However, patients were concerned about feeling safe and free from pain, rather than being in control of their medication. Concerns about the apparatus, overdosing and side effects constrained their sense of being in control. What they did like about PCA was that it removed their need to 'bother' the nurses with requests for pain relief. Thus a technology that is ostensibly designed to benefit patients in fact serves the convenience of staff in addition to effectively reducing the amount of direct interaction between nurses and patients (Salmon & Hall 2004).

Decisions

The idealised formulae of shared decision making and patient-centred medicine have proved hard to map onto the indeterminate and inchoate reality of clinical practice. Decisions are often assumed to be discrete and identifiable events, rather than complex, overlapping, iterative and extended processes (Paterson, Russell & Thorne 2001). Some decisions, once reached, are irreversible. Many, however, involve ongoing critical scrutiny, reappraisal, legitimation, fluctuating commitment and reversal. Often decisions may only be judged retrospectively, after their outcome has become manifest. It is evident that patients carry on the decision making process long after they have left the consultation (Donovan & Blake 1992). What does it mean to say that a decision can be 'shared' or, often, even identified? As we have seen, the etiquette of the consultation dictates that agreement should be displayed, even if this amounts to no more than concealed resistance by the patient. Evaluating the 'quality' of a decision is also a problem (Broadstock & Michie 2000). It is generally assumed that 'good' decisions need to be well informed, but this is not necessarily the case. Neither does it follow that actively involving patients in decision making necessarily results in good decisions (Entwistle & Watt 2004). Analysis of medical decision making tends to assume that actors process information in the course of carefully evaluating alternatives in a thorough and rational manner. The costs and benefits of different options are systematically compared in order to identify the choice which 'maximises expected utility'. Decision aids are generally strongly oriented to providing information to make up the shortfall in patients' knowledge and so extend the processes of cognitive filtering which will facilitate a good decision. However, in the real world, not only is information rarely 'complete' (even for experts), it is only one of many factors influencing decisions, alongside a complex mix of contextual factors, including emotion, aesthetics, social constraints and obligations and personal values and goals (Broadstock & Michie 2000; Pollock 2001). Recently attention has turned to an examination of the processes of naturalistic decision making as these occur spontaneously in real life situations. This reveals the importance of the intuitive processes and heuristic shortcuts that enable people to respond quickly and often effectively to emerging situations of challenge and uncertainty. Broadstock and Michie conclude that although analytic thinking may be appropriate for working through some kinds of problem, the naturalistic decision making paradigm may be more suited to dealing with the intrinsically complex, uncertain and value driven problems which the experience of illness poses (Broadstock & Michie 2000).

Patient-centred medicine and shared decision making have been proposed as a means of overcoming an outmoded and inefficient mode of interaction between patients and health professionals. They are also viewed as powerful levers for increasing professional accountability and improving the quality and efficiency of healthcare. Medical paternalism is widely regarded to be unacceptable in perpetuating patient dependence and passivity and to be directly antithetical to culturally prevailing norms and ideals of citizenship in a consumer society.

> Paternalism is harmful to health because it fosters passivity, sapping self-confidence and undermining people's ability to cope. Paternalistic relationships create and reinforce dependence on health professionals. This in turn breeds resentment on both sides.
>
> Coulter (2002: 107)

Personal autonomy and self-determination are manifest in freedom of choice. Self-reliance, in healthcare as in other areas of behaviour, is taken to be self-evidently good and desirable, and to deliver benefits to the wider society as well as the patient. Makoul identifies self-reliance as a key determinant of involvement in shared decision making (Makoul 1998). In addition to improving individual wellbeing and health outcomes, wider social and economic benefits follow in the form of reduced demand on health services and associated costs.

However well intentioned, it is apparent that patient-centred medicine, shared decision making and concordance are primarily professional and ideological constructs. It is evident that their impact on medical practice and the inter-relationships between patients and health professionals has been limited to date.

The previous chapter reviewed the normative interactional and cultural constraints and functions which bolster lingering inertia in the conduct of medical consultations. The present chapter has discussed the effect of such constructs in increasing the complexity and uncertainty of professional and patient roles, and raised some doubts about the extent to which they correspond in fact with lay preferences or contribute to a demonstrable health gain. We turn now to a further key component of shared decision making in medical consultations: the informed and expert patient.

References

Altiner A, Knauf A, Moebes J, Sielk M and Wilm S (2004) Acute cough: a qualitative analysis of how GPs manage the consultation when patients explicitly or implicitly expect antibiotic prescriptions. *Family Practice*. **21**(5): 500–6.

Barry C, Bradley C, Britten N, Stevenson F and Barber N (2000) Patients' unvoiced agendas in general practice consultations. *BMJ*. **320**: 1246–50.

Barry M, Cherkin D, Chang Y, Fowler F and Skates S (1997) A randomized trial of a multimedia shared decision-making program for men facing a treatment decision for benign prostatic hyperplasia. *Disease Management and Clinical Outcomes*. **1**: 5–14.

Bekker HL, Hewison J and Thornton JG (2003) Understanding why decision aids work: linking process with outcome. *Patient Education and Counselling*. **50**: 323–9.

Bishop FL and Yardley L (2004) Constructing agency in treatment decisions: negotiating responsibility in cancer. *Health*. **8**(4): 465–82.

Bloor MJ and Horobin GW (1975) Conflict and conflict resolution in doctor/patient interactions. In: C Cox and A Mead (eds) *A Sociology of Medical Practice*. Collier-MacMillan, London, pp. 271–84.

Braddock CH, Edwards KA, Hasenberg NM, Laidley TL and Levinson W (1999) Informed decision making in outpatient practice: time to get back to basics. *Journal of the American Medical Association*. **282**: 2313–20.

Britten N (2004) Patients' expectations of consultations. *BMJ*. **328**(21 February): 416–17.

Britten N, Stevenson F, Barry C, Barber N and Bradley C (2000) Misunderstanding in prescribing decisions in general practice: a qualitative study. *BMJ*. **320**: 484–8.

Britten N, Stevenson F, Gafaranga J, Barry C and Bradley C (2004) The expression of aversion to medicines in general practice consultations. *Social Science and Medicine*. **59**: 1495–503.

Broadstock M and Michie S (2000) Processes of patient decision making: theoretical and methodological issues. *Psychology and Health*. **15**: 191–204.

Burkitt Wright E, Holcombe C and Salmon P (2004) Doctors' communication of trust, care, and respect in breast cancer: qualitative study. *BMJ*. **328**(10 April): 864–7.

Butler C, Rollnick S, Pill R, Maggs-Rapport F and Stott N (1998) Understanding the culture of prescribing: qualitative study of general practitioners' and patients' perceptions of antibiotics for sore throats. *BMJ*. **317**: 637–42.

Butler NM, Campion PD and Cox AD (1992) Exploration of doctor and patient agendas in general practice consultations. *Social Science and Medicine*. **35**(9): 1145–55.

Cape J and McCullough Y (1999) Patients' reasons for not presenting emotional problems in general practice consultations. *British Journal of General Practice*. **49**: 875–9.

Charles C, Gafni A and Whelan T (1997) Shared decision-making in the medical encounter: what does it mean? (Or it takes at least two to tango). *Social Science and Medicine*. **44**(5): 681–92.

Charles C, Whelan T and Gafni A (1999) What do we mean by partnership in making decisions about treatment? *BMJ*. **319**.

Charles C, Whelan T, Gafni A, Reyno L and Redko C (1998) Doing nothing is no choice: lay constructions of decision making among women with early stage breast cancer. *Sociology of Health and Illness*. **20**: 71–95.

Chewning B and Wiederholt JB (2003) Concordance in cancer medication management. *Patient Education and Counselling*. **50**: 75–8.

Cockburn J and Pitt S (1997) Prescribing behaviour in general practice: patients' expectations and doctors' perceptions of patients' expectations. *BMJ*. **315**: 520–30.

Cohen H and Britten N (2003) Who decides about prostate cancer treatment? A qualitative study. *Family Practice*. **20**(6): 724–9.

Coulter A (1997) Partnerships with patients: the pros and cons of shared decision-making. *Journal of Health Services Research and Policy*. **2**: 112–21.

Coulter A (2002) *The Autonomous Patient: ending paternalism in medical care*. The Nuffield Trust, London.

Coulter A, Peto V and Doll H (1994) Patients' preferences and general practitioners' decisions in the treatment of menstrual disorders. *Family Practice*. **11**: 67–74.

Cox K, Stevenson F, Britten N and Dundar Y (2004) *A Systematic Review of Communication Between Patients and Health Care Professionals About Medicine-taking and Prescribing*. Medicines Partnership, London.

Coyle J (1999) Exploring the meaning of 'dissatisfaction' with health care: the importance of 'personal identity threat'. *Sociology of Health and Illness*. **21**: 95–124.

de Haes H and Koedoot N (2003) Patient centered decision making in palliative cancer treatment: a world of paradoxes. *Patient Education and Counselling*. **50**: 43–9.

Department of Health (1991) *The Patient's Charter*. Department of Health, London.

Department of Health (1996) *Patient Partnership: building a collaborative strategy*. Department of Health, National Health Service Executive, London.

Department of Health (1998) *In the Public Interest: developing a strategy for public participation in the NHS*. Department of Health NHS Executive.

Department of Health (1999) *Patient and Public Involvement in the New NHS*. Department of Health, London.

Department of Health (2000) *The NHS Plan: a plan for investment, a plan for reform*. Department of Health, London.

Department of Health (2001a) *Involving Patients and the Public in Healthcare: a discussion document*. Department of Health, London.

Department of Health (2001b) *The Expert Patient: a new approach to chronic disease management for the 21st century*. Department of Health, London.

Deyo R (2000) Tell it like it is: patients as partners in medical decision making. *Journal of General Internal Medicine*. **15**: 752–4.

Donovan J and Blake D (1992) Patient non-compliance: deviance or reasoned decision-making? *Social Science and Medicine*. **35**(5): 507–13.

Dowell J (2004) The prescriber's perspective. In: C Bond (ed.) *Concordance: a partnership in medicine taking*. Pharmaceutical Press, London, pp. 49–70.

Dowell J, Jones A and Snadden D (2002) Exploring medication use to seek concordance with 'non-adherent' patients: a qualitative study. *British Journal of General Practice*. **52**: 24–32.

Dowrick C (1999) Uncertainty and responsibility. In: C Dowrick and L Frith (eds) *General Practice and Ethics: uncertainty and responsibility*. Routledge, London, pp. 13–27.

Edwards A and Elwyn G (2001) *Evidence-based Patient Choice: inevitable or impossible?* Oxford University Press, Oxford.

Edwards A, Elwyn G, Smith C, Williams S and Thornton H (2001) Consumers' views of quality in the consultation and their relevance to 'shared decision-making' approaches. *Health Expectations*. **4**(3): 151–61.

Edwards A, Elwyn G and Mulley A (2002) Explaining risks: turning numerical data into meaningful pictures. *BMJ*. **324**: 827–30.

Edwards A, Evans R and Elwyn G (2003) Manufactured but not imported: new directions for research in shared decision making support and skills. *Patient Education and Counselling.* **50**: 33–8.

Elwyn G and Charles C (2001) Shared decision making: the principles and the competences. In: A Edwards and G Elwyn (eds) *Evidence-based Patient Choice: inevitable or impossible?* Oxford University Press, Oxford, pp. 118–43.

Elwyn G, Edwards A, Gwyn R and Grol R (1999a) Towards a feasible model for shared decision making: focus group study with general practitioners. *BMJ.* **319**: 753–6.

Elwyn G, Gwyn R, Edwards A and Grol R (1999b) Is 'shared decision making' feasible in consultations for upper respiratory tract infections? Assessing the influence of antibiotic expectations using discourse analysis. *Health Expectations.* **2**: 105–17.

Elwyn G, Edwards A, Hood K, Robling M, Atwell C, Russell I, Wensing M and Grol R (2004) Achieving involvement: process outcomes from a cluster randomized trial of shared decision making skill development and use of risk communication aids in general practice. *Family Practice.* **21**(4): 337–46.

Elwyn G, Edwards A and Kinnersley P (1999) Shared decision-making in primary care: the neglected second half of the consultation. *British Journal of General Practice.* **49**: 477–82.

Elwyn G, Edwards A, Kinnersley P and Grol R (2000) Shared decision making and the concept of equipoise: the competences of involving patients in healthcare choices. *British Journal of General Practice.* **50**: 892–7.

Entwistle V, Sheldon TA, Sowden A and Watt IS (1998) Evidence informed patient choice, practical issues of involving patients in decisions about health care technologies. *International Journal of Technology Assessment in Health Care.* **14**: 212–25.

Entwistle V, Watt I, Bugge C, Collins S, Drew P, Gilhooly K and Walker A (2002) *Exploring Patient Participation in Decision-making.* Department of Health, London. http://www.healthinpartnership.org/publications/entwistle/entwistle-final.html

Fallowfield L (2001) Participation of patients in decisions about treatment of cancer. *BMJ.* **323**(17 November): 1144.

Fitzpatrick R, Hopkins A and Harvard-Watt (1983) Social dimensions of healing: a longtitudinal study of outcomes of medical management of headaches. *Social Science and Medicine.* **17**: 501–10.

Ford S, Schofield T and Hope T (2002) Barriers to the evidence-based patient choice (EBPC) consultation. *Patient Education and Counselling.* **47**: 179–85.

Frankel S, Ebrahim S and Davey Smith G (2000) The limits to demand for health care. *BMJ.* **321**: 40–5.

Freeman AC and Sweeney K (2001) Why general practitioners do not implement evidence: qualitative study. *BMJ.* **323**(10 November): 1100.

Gafni A, Charles C and Whelan T (1998) The physician–patient encounter: The physician as a perfect agent for the patient versus the informed treatment decision-making model. *Social Science and Medicine.* **47**: 347–54.

Galletari M, Butow PN and Tattersall MHN (2001) Sharing decisions in cancer care. *Social Science and Medicine.* **52**: 1865–78.

Greenfield S, Kaplan SH, Ware JE, Yano EM and Frank HJ (1988) Patients' participation in medical care: effects on blood sugar control and quality of life in diabetes. *Journal of General Internal Medicine.* **3**: 448–57.

Guadagnoli E and Ward P (1998) Patient participation in decision-making. *Social Science and Medicine.* **47**: 329–39.

Gwyn R and Elwyn G (1999) When is a shared decision not (quite) a shared decision? Negotiating preferences in a general practice encounter. *Social Science and Medicine.* **49**: 437–47.

Harrison A and New B (2002) *Public Interest, Private Decisions: health-related research in the UK.* King's Fund, London.

Hogg C (1999) *Patients, Power and Politics: from patients to citizens.* Sage Publications, London.

Holmes-Rovner M, Valade D, Orlowski C, Draus C and Nabozny-Valerio K (2000)

Implementing shared decision making in routine practice: barriers and opportunities. *Health Expectations.* **3**: 182–91.

Hope T (1996) *Evidence Based Patient Choice.* King's Fund, London.

Howitt A and Armstrong D (1999) Implementing evidence based medicine in general practice: audit and qualitative study of antithrombotic treatment for atrial fibrillation. *BMJ.* **318**: 1324–7.

Ingelfinger FJ (1980) Arrogance. *New England Journal of Medicine.* **303**(26): 1507–11.

Kaplan SH, Greenfield S and Ware JE (1989) Impact of the doctor–patient relationship on the outcomes of chronic disease. In: M Stewart and DL Roter (eds) *Communicating with Medical Patients.* Sage Publications, London.

Kenny P, Quine S, Shiell A and Cameron S (1999) Participation in treatment decision-making by women with early stage breast cancer. *Health Expectations.* **2**: 159–68.

Kettunen T, Poskiparta M, Liimatainen L, Sjogren A and Karhila P (2001) Taciturn patients in health counselling at a hospital: passive recipients or active participators? *Qualitative Health Research.* **11**(3): 399–410.

Little P, Dorward M, Warner G, Stephens K, Senior J and Moore M (2004) Importance of patient pressure and perceived pressure and perceived medical need for investigations, referral, and prescribing in primary care: nested observational study. *BMJ.* **328**: 444.

Little P, Everitt H, Williamson I, Warner G, Moore M, Gould C, Ferrier K and Payne S (2001) Observational study of effect of patient centredness and positive approach on outcomes of general practice consultations. *BMJ.* **323**: 908–11.

Little P, Gould C, Williamson I, Warner G, Gantley M and Kinmonth A L (1999) Clinical and psychosocial predictors of illness duration from randomised controlled trial of prescribing strategies for sore throat. *BMJ.* **319**: 736–7.

Lupton D (1997) Consumerism, reflexivity and the medical encounter. *Social Science and Medicine.* **45**(3): 373–81.

Makoul G (1998) Perpetuating passivity: reliance and reciprocal determinism in physician–patient interaction. *Journal of Health Communication.* **3**: 233–59.

Marvel MK, Epstein RM, Flowers K and Beckman HB (1999) Soliciting the patient's agenda: have we improved? *Journal of the American Medical Association.* **281**(3): 283–7.

Maseide P (1991) Possibly abusive, often benign, and always necessary. On power and domination in medical practice. *Sociology of Health and Illness.* **13**(4): 545–61.

May C and Mead N (1998) Patient-centredness: A history. In: L Frith and C Dowrick (eds) *Ethical Issues in General Practice: uncertainty and responsibility.* Routledge, London, pp. 76–90.

Maynard DW (1991) Interaction and asymmetry in clinical discourse. *American Journal of Sociology.* **97**(2): 448–95.

McKevitt C and Morgan M (1997) Anomalous patients: the experiences of doctors with an illness. *Sociology of Health and Illness.* **19**(5): 644–67.

McKinley RK and Middleton JF (1999) What do patients want from doctors? Content analysis of written patient agendas for the consultation. *British Journal of General Practice.* **49**: 796–800.

McPherson K (1994) The best and the enemy of the good: randomised controlled trials, uncertainty, and assessing the role of patient choice in medical decision making. *Journal of Epidemiology and Community Health.* **48**: 6–15.

Mead N and Bower P (2002) Patient-centred consultations and outcomes in primary care: a review of the literature. *Patient Education and Counselling.* **48**: 51–61.

Misselbrook D and Armstrong D (2001) Patients' responses to risk information about the benefits of treating hypertension. *British Journal of General Practice.* **51**: 276–9.

NHSCRD (2000) Informing, communicating and sharing decisions with people who have cancer. *Effective Health Care.* **6**(6): 1–8.

O'Connor A and Edwards A (2001) The role of decision aids in promoting evidence-based patient choice. In: A Edwards and G Elwyn (eds) *Evidence-Based Patient Choice: inevitable or impossible?* Oxford University Press, Oxford, pp. 220–42.

O'Connor A, Rostom A, Fiset V, Tetroe J, Entwistle V, Llewellyn-Thomas H, Holmes-Rovner M, Barry M and Jones J (1999) Decision aids for patients facing health treatment or screening decisions: systematic review. *BMJ.* **319**(18 September): 731–4.

Patel HRH, Mirsadraee S and Emberton M (2003) The patient's dilemma: prostate cancer treatment choices. *Journal of Urology.* **169**(March): 828–33.

Paterson BL, Russell C and Thorne S (2001) Critical analysis of everyday self-care decision making in chronic illness. *Journal of Advanced Nursing.* **35**(3): 335–41.

Pollock K (2001) 'I've not asked him, you see, and he's not said': understanding lay explanatory models of illness is a prerequisite for concordant consultations. *International Journal of Pharmacy Practice.* **9**(2): 105–18.

Pollock K, Grime J, Baker E and Mantala K (2004) Meeting the information needs of psychiatric inpatients: staff and patient perspectives. *Journal of Mental Health.* **13**(4): 389–401.

Protheroe J, Fahey T, Montgomery A and Peters T (2000) The impact of patients' preferences on the treatment of atrial fibrillation: observational study of patient based decision analysis. *BMJ.* **320**: 1380–4.

Punamaki R-L and Kokko SJ (1995) Content and predictors of consultation experiences among Finnish primary care patients. *Social Science and Medicine.* **40**: 231–43.

Quill TE and Brody H (1996) Physician recommendations and patient autonomy: finding a balance between physician power and patient choice. *Annals of Internal Medicine.* **125**(9): 763–9.

Radley A (1996) The critical moment: time, information and medical expertise in the experience of patients receiving coronary bypass surgery. In: S Williams and M Calnan (eds) *Modern Medicines: lay perspectives and experiences.* UCL Press, London, pp. 118–38.

Rees Jones I, Berney L, Kelly M, Doyal L, Griffiths C, Feder G, Hillier S, Rowlands G and Curtis S (2004) Is patient involvement possible when decisions involve scarce resources? A qualitative study of decision-making in primary care. *Social Science and Medicine.* **59**(1): 93-102.

Reis S, Hermoni D, Livingstone P and Borkan J (2002) Case report of paroxysmal atrial fibrillation and anticoagulation. *BMJ.* **325**(2 November):1018–20.

Rosenberg SG (1976) Patient education: an educator's view. In: DL Sackett and R Haynes (eds) *Compliance with Therapeutic Regimes.* Johns Hopkins University Press, Baltimore, pp. 93–9.

Roter DL (2000) The medical visit context of treatment decision-making and the therapeutic relationship. *Health Expectations.* **3**: 17–25.

Roter DL, Stewart M, Putnam SM, Lipkin M, Stiles W and Inui TS (1997) Communication patterns of primary care physicians. *Journal of the American Medical Association.* **277**(4): 350–6.

RPSGB (1997) *From Compliance to Concordance, Achieving Shared Goals in Medicine Taking.* Royal Pharmaceutical Society of Great Britain, London.

Salkeld G, Solomon M, Short L and Butow PN (2004) A matter of trust – patient's views on decision-making in colorectal cancer. *Health Expectations.* **7**: 104–14.

Salmon P and Hall GM (2003) Patient empowerment and control: a psychological discourse in the service of medicine. *Social Science and Medicine.* **57**(10): 1969-80.

Salmon P and Hall GM (2004) Patient empowerment of the emperor's new clothes. *Journal of the Royal Society for Medicine.* **97**: 53–6.

Salmon P and Manyande A (1996) Good patients cope with their pain: postoperative analgesia and nurses' perceptions of their patients' pain. *Pain.* **68**: 63–8.

Schwartz RK, Soumeris B and Ajorn J (1989) Physician motivations for non-scientific drug prescribing. *Social Science and Medicine.* **28**(6): 577–82.

Silverman D (1987a) Coercive interpretation of the clinic: the social constitution of the

Down's Syndrome child. In: D Silverman (ed.) *Communication and Medical Practice: social relations in the clinic*. Sage Publications, London.

Silverman D (1987b) *Communication and Medical Practice: social relations in the clinic*. Sage Publications, London.

Stapleton H, Kirkham M and Thomas G (2002) Qualitative study of evidence based leaflets in maternity care. *BMJ*. **324**(16 March): 639.

Stevenson F, Barry C, Britten N, Barber N and Bradley C (2000) Doctor–patient communication about drugs: the evidence for shared decision making. *Social Science and Medicine*. **50**: 829–40.

Stewart M (1995) Effective physician–patient communication and health outcomes: a review. *Canadian Medical Association Journal*. **152**: 1423–33.

Strull WM, Lo B and Charles G (1984) Do patients want to participate in medical decision making? *Journal of the American Medical Association*. **252**: 2990–4.

Thorne S, Ternulf Nyhlin K and Paterson BL (2000) Attitudes toward patient expertise in chronic illness. *International Journal of Nursing Studies*. **37**: 303–11.

Tomlin Z, Humphrey C and Rogers S (1999) General practitioners' perceptions of effective health care. *BMJ*. **318**: 1532–5.

Towle A and Godolphin W (1999) Framework for teaching and learning informed shared decision making. *BMJ*. **319**(18 September): 766–71.

Veldhuis M, Wigersma L and Okkes I (1998) Deliberate departures from good general practice: a study of motives among Dutch general practitioners. *British Journal of General Practice*. **48**: 1833–6.

Weiss M (2004) Educational perspectives on concordance. In: C Bond (ed.) *Concordance: a partnership in medicine taking*. Pharmaceutical Press, London, pp. 91–118.

Weiss M and Scott D (1997) Whose rationality? A qualitative analysis of general practitioners' prescribing. *Pharmaceutical Journal*. **259**: 339–41.

Wennberg JE, Barry MJ, Fowler FJ and Mulley A (1993) Outcomes research, PORTs and health care reform. *Annals New York Academy of Sciences*. **703**: 52–62.

Werner A and Malterud K (2003) It is hard work behaving as a credible patient: encounters between women with chronic pain and their doctors. *Social Science and Medicine*. **57**: 1409–19.

Werner A, Widding Isaksen L and Malterud K (2004) 'I am not the kind of woman who complains of everything': Illness stories on self and shame in women with chronic pain. *Social Science and Medicine*. **59**: 1035–45.

West P (1976) The physician and the management of childhood epilepsy. In: M Wadsworth and D Robinson (eds) *Studies in Everyday Medical Life*. Martin Robertson, London.

Williams S and Calnan M (1996a) Modern medicine and the lay populace: theoretical perspectives and methodological issues. In: S Williams and M Calnan (eds) *Modern Medicine: lay perspectives and experiences*. UCL Press, London, pp. 2–25.

Williams S and Calnan M (1996b) Modern medicine and the lay populace in late modernity. In: S Williams and M Calnan (eds) *Modern Medicine: lay perspectives and experience*. UCL Press, London, pp. 256–64.

Chapter Eight

The informed and expert patient

Introduction

The highly educated populations of modern industrial societies have unprece-dented and virtually unlimited access to specialist information on just about any subject that takes their interest. Health and illness have become topics of particular social and personal concern and the focus of a vast industry producing materials giving advice and instruction about how to preserve health, in the first instance, and deal with illness in the second. Education is viewed as an important lever in the general reduction of social and economic inequality. The steady erosion of the professional monopoly of expert medical knowledge is seen as a means of overriding the entrenched paternalism of clinical practice and reducing the structured asymmetry of medical consultations. Democratisation of relation-ships between doctors and patients is regarded as intrinsically desirable in an aspirationally meritocratic and egalitarian society. Within the research and policy spheres it is also favoured as a means of increasing professional accountability and improving the quality and efficiency of healthcare. The provision of comprehen-sive and good quality information to patients is viewed as essential to their involvement in shared decision making about treatment and the development of patient-centred medicine as a central goal of current health policy (Coulter 2002a; Makoul, Arntson & Schofield 1995). Nevertheless, the acquisition and practical application of lay specialist knowledge in medical consultations remains a source of tension and difficulty in the relationships between patients and professionals. More generally, the issue of how expert knowledge is processed by individuals and distributed within society requires further exploration and analysis.

Professional interest in patient education originated in the 1970s, with the discovery, and consequent association, of patient ignorance and widespread non-compliance in medicine taking (*see* Chapter 2). Much effort went into producing information materials as a means of remedying the patient deficit assumed to impede the accurate and effective compliance with medical instructions. It soon became apparent, however, that information by itself did not do much to improve compliance (Haynes 1976; Haynes 1979). Early compliance researchers made clear from the outset not only that the onus should be on professionals to communicate more effectively with patients (Ley 1982; Ley & Spelman 1967), but also that compliance was unethical if it was not based on properly informed consent (Haynes & Sackett 1979; Sackett 1976). The establishment of informed consent as a basic right is a precondition for the exercise of patient autonomy (Sullivan 2003). Roter expresses this point forcefully:

> The boundaries of autonomy and paternalism are negotiated through the determination of how much information, with what level of detail, given when, under what circumstances, in whose language, and in what context. As a result of the great variability in patients' ability to negotiate the medical dialogue, ethicists have identified protection from verbal coercion with almost universal regard as a necessary and important element of civilized and enlightened medical care.
>
> Roter (2000: 19)*

The requirements for informed consent remain unclear, and probably are not often achieved (Makoul, Arntson & Schofield 1995; Roter 2000; Rycroft-Malone *et al.* 2001; Sitzia & Wood 1997). However, even as an aspiration, the principle that treatment should only proceed with the individual's full understanding and agreement has been an important spur to the development and provision of patient information. It also presents a challenge to medical paternalism in legitimising patient defined outcomes and prioritising these over clinically derived criteria for evaluating interventions (Sullivan 2003).

Recognition of the need for informed consent is based in ethical concerns and the principle of autonomy which concedes to the individual an inviolable right to determine what happens to his body (Towle & Godolphin 1999). It has been strengthened by the development of increasingly powerful medical technologies and treatments, and the awareness of their power to harm as well as help (Asscher, Parr & Whitmarsh 1995). A substantial proportion of the population is now prescribed powerful drugs on a long-term basis to ameliorate the effects of chronic and degenerative diseases. These have become the price of medical and socio-economic success in overcoming acute infections and extending lives affected by conditions which would formerly have proved quickly fatal. The trade-off between risk and benefit of such interventions is often finely balanced. As was discussed in the previous chapter, treatment decisions frequently involve a consideration of personal values and goals which are particular to the individual patient. While such decisions are influenced by many factors, including emotion, aesthetics and trust, information is clearly an important component.

Professionals have become sensitive to the need to provide patients with comprehensive information as a means of forestalling litigation after patients suffer harm from treatment. Infamous cases of medical negligence or malpractice, such as the retention of body parts at the Alder Hey Children's Hospital in Liverpool (www.rlcinquiry.org.uk/) and the high mortality rate among children undergoing heart surgery at the Bristol Royal Infirmary (www.bristol-inquiry.org.uk/), have heightened the moral case for greater professional transparency. They also reveal the adverse consequences of poor communication, medical paternalism and the exclusion of patients from direct and active involvement in decisions and processes of care (Coulter 2002a; Department of Health 2002a; Roter 2000; Sitzia & Wood 1997). The Bristol Inquiry report fully endorsed the policy of developing patient-centred medical practice. Many of its recommendations are for improvements in patient information, involvement and communication with staff. Patient education and engagement is accorded a role in the process of clinical governance and maintaining high standards of medical practice (Department of Health 2002a).

* Roter DL (2000) Reproduced with permission from Blackwell Publishing, Oxford.

Modern conceptions of citizenship are rooted in the principles of individualism and autonomy (Corrigan 2003). These are expressed in the exercise of choice and underpinned by the development of a personal competence and efficacy which frequently demand a high degree of expertise. Expert knowledge (about health and other subjects) increasingly comes to be taken up as part of popular 'common sense', and even to constitute a cultural resource for the *explanation* of illness as a form of misfortune (Kangas 2002). Consumerism is both a manifestation as well as a stimulus to the free expression of personal choice. The convergence of commercial and government campaigns promoting the message that health depends on styles of living which can be bought and chosen has resulted in health itself increasingly being fashioned as a basic competence of the autonomous individual. Such messages, of course, fly in the face of reality: a substantial proportion of an increasingly ageing population experience long-term management of chronic disease as the norm.

The burden of chronic disease resulting from the continuing extension of average life expectancy in the developed nations could more appropriately be read as a sign of social and economic success rather than personal failure. The continuing prevalence of the patient defect model is well illustrated at the present time by the government's policy commitment to helping individuals to 'choose' health, mainly through the adoption of a prudent lifestyle (Department of Health 2003). This is the latest and most explicit expression of an authoritarian 'healthism' which has been developing over the last several decades (Armstrong 1995; Crawford 1977; Fitzgerald 1994). Crawford (2004) gives an analysis of the contradictory effects of the relentless production and consumption of information about health and illness. This heightens, rather than reduces, a sense of anxiety about personal risk and vulnerability in postmodern society which is pervasive and inescapable (Beck 1992; Bellaby 2001; Vuckovic & Nichter 1997). Knowledge has a double edge, just as easily heightening uncertainty and risk as conveying a sense of understanding and control. Awareness of risk confers responsibility. Like it or not, the modern citizen is becoming obligated to perform an unprecedented amount of routine health maintenance and illness management.

Knowledge is an integral part of that involvement, a requirement for informed consent and active involvement in shared decision making. However, as we saw in the previous chapter, consumerism seems to have made little headway in the consulting room. Interaction between patient and health professionals remains governed by a bureaucratic format which serves to limit the disclosure and free exchange of information. People vary widely in their desire for information or shared decision making. However, dilemmas arise for the informed, or information-seeking, patient. The display or discussion of knowledge by patients is often circumscribed by the assumption that it signifies a criticism of the doctor, or challenge to his expertise (Beach *et al.* 2005; Cohen & Britten 2003; Leydon *et al.* 2000). The inability of highly educated and increasingly well informed patients to reveal their knowledge in medical encounters, *or to have this acknowledged as legitimate* by staff (Thorne, Ternulf Nyhlin & Paterson 2000), illustrates the distance that still remains between policy goals and the reality of routine practice. It also highlights the extent to which professional culture has successfully resisted change and the real world constraints which continue to confound the realisation of genuine informed consent.

The routine provision of high quality information to patients is seen to be a prerequisite for informed consent, shared decision making and patient-centred medicine. Nevertheless, it is hard to know how much information individuals actually need or want in any particular context. The frustration caused by inadequate information, or the inability to share and discuss this with professionals, may be matched by the anxiety and uncertainty resulting from excess. Just as patients do not always want the responsibility of shared decision making (*see* Chapter 7), they may not feel the need to access specialist information about illness and treatment. Knowledge is conventionally perceived to be 'empowering'. In practice, things are less straightforward. Knowledge may become a burden, and where it is seen to be obligatory, an imposition. Patients' expressed desire for information may vary according to context. It may depend, for example, on whether or not they are healthy when considering the question and, if not, on the nature of the problem and whether they are acutely, seriously or chronically ill. People's actual desire for information may correspond to a greater or lesser extent with their expressed desire. However, it is more likely to be discovered in the course of engaging with the contingencies of illness, rather than persist as a fixed and unchanging attribute. Many motives and interests lie behind the campaign for patient education. Alongside an ideological commitment to patient autonomy, shared decision making and improved experience of being a patient are more pragmatic concerns about redistributing cost and the responsibility of healthcare.

Patient information

The patient's right to receive information about treatment was formally recognised in the Patient Charter of 1991, and reinforced and extended in a series of government publications throughout the ensuing decade (Department of Health 1991, 1996, 1998, 1999b, 2001a, 2001b, 2001c, 2002a). These documents recognised that adequate information is a basic entitlement of patients. They also emphasised its positive impact as an enabling factor in disease prevention and reduction. Since 1992 pharmaceutical manufacturers in Europe have been obliged to include a patient information leaflet with all packs of prescription medicines. These, along with much institutionally sourced information materials, have been widely criticised for being user-unfriendly and reflecting commercial and professional concerns and preoccupations instead of being oriented to the expressed needs and preferences of patients. When patients are involved in evaluating and developing patient-centred materials, the discrepancies between the lay and professional perspective of what constitutes 'good' information become readily apparent (Coulter, Entwistle & Gilbert 1998; Crawford & Kessel 1999; Dickinson, Raynor & Duman 2001; Grime & Pollock 2004; Hughes, Whittlesea & Luscombe 2002; Kennedy, Robinson & Rogers 2003; Raynor & Britten 2001; Rose 2001).

Dixon-Woods identifies two separate discourses in her critical analysis of patient information materials (Dixon-Woods 2001). Rapidly widening public access to specialised information has begun to undermine the professional monopoly of expert knowledge which has been an important prop in maintaining medical authority. However, much of the published material most readily available within the public domain remains the product of the dominant biomedical discourse. This largely ignores the patient perspective and seeks to frame information as a means of securing compliance with medical regimes.

Patient autonomy is discounted, since the patient is regarded as basically ignorant and incompetent. In this context, to the extent that the biomedical discourse takes account of, or recognises, the patient view, it is generally as a tactic to engineer compliance, and displace the 'misconceptions' which cause patients to deviate from following professional advice (Horne & Weinman 2004). (Appropriately) informed patients are considered more likely to cooperate with treatment. Within the biomedical discourse patient choices and values, especially concerns about how illness and treatment impact on quality of life, are not considered, nor is there much recognition of entitlement to information as a basic right (Crawford & Kessel 1999; Rose 2001). These are, however, central concerns of the second, and still much less influential, discourse which Dixon-Woods identifies relating to patient empowerment. In effect, and notwithstanding decades of research critiquing medical paternalism, and over 10 years of policy commitment to increasing patient involvement in healthcare, the biomedical discourse still predominates. For many professionals, patient-centred medicine amounts to little more than patients' capacity to benefit from instruction, and concordance has become merely another, more acceptable, term for compliance (Heath 2003).

Verbal information

Dissatisfaction with the quality and provision of patient information is widely reported (Coulter, Entwistle & Gilbert 1998; Coulter, Entwistle & Gilbert 1999; Ley 1997; Ley & Spelman 1967; NHSCRD 2000; Skelton 2001) and has been a particular issue in the area of mental illness (Campbell, Cobb & Darton 1998; Cobb, Darton & Kiran 2001; Rogers, Pilgrim & Lacey 1993; Rose 2001). Nearly half (45%) of the 215 patients interviewed in the Sainsbury Centre survey said that they had not had enough information about their illness or treatment. In contrast, staff considered this to be a problem for only 9% of these cases (Sainsbury Centre for Mental Health 1998). Rose *et al.* also found that half of the mental health service users they surveyed felt they were inadequately informed about their treatment. A third felt that they were being over-medicated, with a consequently damaging effect on their quality of life. This report indicated that staff rarely consulted users in discussing medication. As a consequence, users remained uninvolved in decisions about care and treatment. There was, however, a significant association between reported involvement and receipt of treatment information by patients and their expressed satisfaction with care (Rose 2001).

Many doctors still consider themselves to be the principal and most appropriate source of information, and continue to be regarded as such by many patients (Cotten & Gupta 2004; Henwood *et al.* 2003; Makoul, Arntson & Schofield 1995; McGrath 1999; Skelton 2001). However, it is evident that professionals tend to underestimate the amount and range of information patients want about their treatment and that the information given to patients in medical consultations, particularly about treatment options and prescribed medicines, is frequently cursory and inadequate (Coulter, Entwistle & Gilbert 1998; Nair *et al.* 2002; Rycroft-Malone *et al.* 2001; Stevenson *et al.* 2000). In their study of communication about medicines in general practice consultations Stevenson *et al.* found that GPs frequently failed to identify a newly prescribed drug by name, sometimes omitted details of correct dosage and often omitted any mention of possible side effects. They made assumptions about patient preferences and need for information without checking them. Patients' deference to medical authority meant that such attributions went unchallenged and uncorrected (Stevenson *et al.* 2000). Makoul *et al.* found not only that the GPs in their study tended to overestimate the amount of information they gave patients, and the extent to which they discussed treatment issues, but so also did the patients. Nearly a quarter of their respondents left the consultation with an 'illusion of competence', stating that they had been adequately informed and even discussed important topics relating to their medication which the taped record showed had not actually taken place (Makoul, Arntson & Schofield 1995).

Professional framing and selective disclosure is a significant issue in the provision of information in medical consultations. Far from being objective and neutral providers of information, doctors habitually select what they feel it is appropriate for patients to know and will encourage them to comply with treatment (Elwyn *et al.* 1999b; Garlick 2003; Silverman 1987; Stapleton, Kirkham & Thomas 2002). They may also be concerned to provide reassurance and encouragement. Steering patients – intentionally or otherwise – in a predetermined direction constitutes a form of censorship which forestalls their ability to make informed and autonomous decisions about treatment. Smith and Henderson found that doctors who assessed themselves as providing a lot of information about treatment side effects to psychiatric patients were actually quite selective about which of these they chose to disclose (Elwyn *et al.* 1999b; Silverman 1987; Smith & Henderson 2000). Doctors' withholding of negative information, especially about side effects, is often related to concerns about non-compliance (McGrath 1999; Nair *et al.* 2002). In fact available evidence suggests that information does not discourage patients from taking their medicines, though it may increase their insight and satisfaction with treatment (Chaplin & Kent 1998; MacPherson, Jerrom & Hughes 1996).

Textual information

Given the risk of bias and framing in professionally presented information, it is important that patients can access good quality and independent alternatives. However, analysis of printed texts reveals their tendency to replicate the same limitations and prejudices (Coulter, Entwistle & Gilbert 1998; Coulter, Entwistle & Gilbert 1999; Garlick 2003; Grime & Pollock 2004; Thornton, Edwards & Baum 2003). Many information materials are produced by professionals or written within a conventional biomedical framework of knowledge. They tend to reproduce the professional view of what patients want or need to know, and to be oriented to encouraging patients to follow their doctors' advice uncritically. In an influential review Coulter *et al.* concluded that available materials contained numerous inaccuracies and misleading statements, rarely attributed sources or cited supporting evidence, and often failed to include details of publication date, sponsorship or authorship. They were often patronising and elementary, failed to acknowledge uncertainty or risk attached to different treatments, and to present these in an unrealistically optimistic light. Far from 'empowering' consumers, much of the available patient information literature was judged likely to *reduce* patients' capacity for shared decision making and informed consent (Coulter, Entwistle & Gilbert 1998; Raynor & Britten 2001).

As well as quality of content, access and distribution are also important. Especially in institutional settings, patients are largely dependent on staff to make information available. Pollock *et al.* found that patients on acute psychiatric wards were rarely able to access written information about their medicines. Leaflets were held on the wards, but were generally kept out of reach of patients, who consequently remained unaware of their existence. The most usual response of staff to specific requests from patients was to give out a copy of the patient information leaflet relating to individual drugs: these were not routinely made available to patients while they were on the wards. The nursing staff, in particular, more or less deliberately sought to position themselves as intermediaries controlling patients' access to information. They were more likely to undertake investigation of an issue raised by patients, and then report back their findings, rather than facilitate patients' access to independent sources of information (Pollock *et al.* 2004). Stapleton, Kirkham & Thomas reported a similar finding in the very different context of antenatal clinics. Once again, staff withheld leaflets from patient access if they disapproved of the content or felt that they described options that they were unable to supply. Here, also, staff tended to make assumptions about patient capacity and desire for involvement in decision making. The researchers concluded that, despite an expressed commitment to patients' exercise of free choice, professional strategies of information management were in fact successfully oriented to securing informed compliance. Women's trust in their professional advisors largely ensured their acceptance of choices that were effectively being taken for them. Normative clinical procedures and practice were established through the preferences of consultants, which junior staff felt unable to challenge. They were consequently unable to support women who expressed preferences for management strategies which were at variance with standard clinic routines (Stapleton, Kirkham & Thomas 2002).

Patients who regard health professionals as their principal sources of information are unlikely to receive a very full or objective presentation. This does not mean they are necessarily dissatisfied with the situation, or that their needs are unmet. However, within the very wide spectrum of desire, it is evident that many patients want more information than they get. Knowledgeable patients tend to make different choices from those who are not (Misselbrook & Armstrong 2001; Protheroe *et al.* 2000; Wennberg *et al.* 1993). Good information about available treatment options and their risks and side effects, in particular, is necessary for the exercise of choice. In pursuit of increased compliance, professionals overlook the extent to which medical decisions are determined by subjective values rather than objective clinical criteria.

Coulter *et al.* (1998) list some of the processes which good information can support and so contribute to improved healthcare delivery. These include: disease prevention, a knowledge and understanding of what is wrong and what can be done about it, including the extent of available resources and processes and intended outcomes of healthcare, the promotion of self-care, the reduction of anxiety and the evaluation of treatment choices. Respondents in Pollock *et al.*'s study of information needs among psychiatric inpatients referred to a wide range of information applications. These included understanding what was wrong, the justification and outcomes of tests and treatments, likely illness prognosis, promotion of self-care, awareness of services and self-help support, reassurance, coping strategies, a basis for informing others about what was wrong, legitimising help seeking, and enabling access to further information (Pollock *et al.* 2004). Mental health users responding to MIND's most recent yellow card scheme for reporting adverse drug effects expressed the need for information about their medicines so that they could understand what they were taking and why, how the drugs acted and possible side effects, including effects on the brain and the risks of harm from long-term treatment, length of treatment, withdrawal symptoms and how to stop treatment, other users' experience of taking the drugs and new types of medication, and non-drug therapeutic options, including alternative and talking therapies (Cobb, Darton & Kiran 2001).

Good quality patient information materials would be centred on patients' expressed concerns and defined needs. They would be oriented to the realities and problems of daily living and optimising quality of life rather than professional conceptions of what patients ought to know (Garlick 2003; Grime & Pollock 2004; Nair *et al.* 2002). Compliance does not feature as a salient issue for patients. Independently produced and accurate information is required for patients to become well informed and in a position to exercise genuine choice. Proponents of Evidence-Based Patient Choice (EBPC) call for patient information to be drawn from the same evidence base that is available to professionals (Edwards & Elwyn 2001; Hope 1996). The patient's current double bind is that since they cannot easily access adequate information it is difficult to acquire the knowledge necessary for professional acceptance of their competence to engage in shared decision making about treatment.

Patient expertise

Professional resistance to the idea of patient expertise constitutes a significant obstacle in path of patient-centred medicine (Faulkener & Thomas 2002; Fox, Ward & O'Rourke 2005; Thorne, Ternulf Nyhlin & Paterson 2000). Elwyn *et al.* comment on the 'unchallenged irritation' expressed by general practitioners towards the idea of the 'informed patient' (Edwards & Elwyn 2001; Elwyn *et al.* 1999a; Hope 1996). The stereotype of the patient entering the consulting room clutching a printout of information downloaded from the internet is one manifestation of this. This negative attribution features prominently in contemporary medical folklore, despite lack of evidence that it is a frequent occurrence (Budtz & Witt 2002; Henwood *et al.* 2003; Malone *et al.* 2004). Thorne *et al.* found that, even in situations when they had no expertise to offer, health professionals maintained their assumption of superior competence when dealing with patients who were genuinely expert in their sophisticated management of diabetes. A particular point of conflict arose over insulin dosage during periods of hospital care. Staff assumed their judgement to be superior to that of patients who had successfully managed their diabetes over many years. Patients' awareness that their expertise and competence were discounted impaired their sense of trust and reduced the therapeutic potential of their relationships with staff. Professional control was perpetuated through the usual techniques of interactional dominance involving dismissal, ridicule and the discrediting of patient contributions. It is noteworthy that even these expert patients often felt too vulnerable and dependent on staff for access to healthcare resources and treatment to risk jeopardising their goodwill by taking a more assertive or confrontational stance (Thorne, Ternulf Nyhlin & Paterson 2000).

Following a review of the evidence, the National Institute of Mental Health (NIMH) acknowledged the significant benefits of self-help interventions (typically based on cognitive behaviour therapy approaches) for people with mental health problems. Nevertheless, the report advises caution: because of the (remote) risk that such materials may be used inappropriately or deter people from seeking *proper* professional help, they should not be used outside of a planned package of care including professional support. Additionally, it is suggested that professionals should become actively involved in providing guidance and support to voluntary sector agencies and self-help groups in their use of self-help materials (NIMHE 2003). The assumption here is that self-help is clearly an inferior second best with at most a supplementary role to professional care. The authority of established expertise is mirrored in the hierarchy of knowledge. Professionally authored sources of patient information are accorded greater credibility and status than those produced within the lay and alternative sectors. This is in stark contrast to lay proponents of self-help, particularly in the area of mental health, who view the acquisition of patient expertise as both a necessary compensation to the inadequacies of clinical care, and a means of resisting the coercive and damaging effects of professional medicine (Barnes & Shardlow 1996; Crossley & Crossley 2001; Shapiro, Mosqueda & Botros 2003; Tennant 2002). The normative role of deferential patient inhibits the display and formal recognition of patient expertise and negates the legitimacy of lay knowledge (Heritage 1997). The self-help movement initiative centres on a contest over power not just to possess, but also to display and legitimise knowledge.

Notwithstanding their formal acceptance of the principles of patient involvement, in the end for many professionals it is just not possible to accept the core principle of concordance that the informed patient's values and preferences for treatment take precedence over those of professionals (Horne & Weinman 2004). This resistance is rationalised in several ways. Lack of confidence in patient competence underlies a widespread concern not only that patients will make bad and inappropriate decisions about treatment, but also that promoting patient choice will open the floodgates of unbridled demand. Prescribers are viewed as having a duty to regulate the equitable distribution of scarce resources, and to prevent individual demand from damaging collective interests (Appleby, Harrison & Devlin 2003; Horne & Weinman 2004). These, usually hypothetical, arguments about the irrational or unreasonable patient are not supported by the empirical evidence reviewed above, which points to the tendency for informed patients to show greater risk aversion and a more conservative approach to treatment than their doctors (Misselbrook & Armstrong 2001; Protheroe *et al.* 2000; Wennberg *et al.* 1993). Indeed, Coulter suggests that greater involvement of patients in choosing treatment may *reduce* rather than increase demand – and cost – within the health service (Coulter 2002b).

A slightly different point to the concern that patients will tend to choose extravagantly and expensively relates to the conviction that the failure of patients to accept their doctors' recommendations will necessarily have an adverse effect on outcome. This view presumes that the acceptance of patient preferences over clinical judgement is likely to conflict with the professional duty of care (Horne & Weinman 2004). It assumes the innate superiority of professional over lay decision making, and that patient compliance is necessary to optimise healthcare outcomes. Professional incapacity to trust patients to choose wisely is still widespread. From this perspective the contribution of concordance is merely to widen professional awareness of the importance of patient beliefs as a determinant of health behaviour, including medicine taking. This enables a more effective professional response to the correction of the 'misconceptions' which lead to patients' failure to comply with medical treatment (Horne & Weinman 2004). This position remains oblivious to the evidence reviewed above of the uncertainty and ineffectiveness of much medical practice, the considerable harm it causes patients, or the extent to which decisions – whether made by patient or professional – are driven by a complex mixture of rationality and emotion (Heath 2003). There is no acknowledgement here of the importance of the *exchange* of understandings between patients and professionals, or that the professional might have something to learn from the patient's experience and judgement. On the contrary, the expert patient tends to be regarded as demanding and unreasonable. The formal professional commitment to concordance and greater patient involvement has not often been accompanied by an appreciation of what this actually entails, or its considerable implications for practice. 'Empowerment' is accepted and widely understood as a more efficient means to the end of securing the goal of compliance. This tension between the drive to increase patient choice and self-reliance and the tenacious professional commitment to compliance remains a major obstacle to the development of concordance (Fox, Ward & O'Rourke 2005; Misselbrook 2001; Thorne, Ternulf Nyhlin & Paterson 2000).

The expert patient

In contrast to professional caution and resistance, the notion of the expert patient has been enthusiastically endorsed by policy makers as a central component in chronic disease management and in modernising the national health service through the development of patient-centred medicine (Department of Health 1999b, 2001b; Donaldson 2003).

> The expert patient programme is one of the best examples of how a true partnership between the public and health professionals can be formed. If successful it will slow, arrest, or possibly even reverse the progression of the chronic diseases of thousands of patients. It will give those affected the power to manage their conditions more effectively.
>
> Donaldson (2003: 1279)*

The expert patient initiative is based on the work of Kate Lorig and colleagues in Canada with the aim of helping sufferers of chronic disease and pain cope more effectively with their illness and symptoms (Lorig *et al.* 1994; Lorig 2000). Self-management programmes (SMPs) aim to help patients improve, rather than eliminate, the enduring symptoms of chronic illness. However, the goal extends beyond symptom management to the achievement of increased self-esteem and improved quality of life (Lorig *et al.* 1994; Lorig 2000). The key feature of SMPs is that patients are trained to deliver structured programmes of active self-management techniques to groups of other patients. The five core

* Donaldson L (2003) Reproduced with permission from the BMJ Publishing Group.

skills of self-management are problem solving, decision making, resource utilisation, formation of a patient–professional partnership and taking action. These correspond closely to the goals of concordance. Expert patients are also increasingly used in professional education programmes to provide insights into the patient perspective of living with chronic illness. This is recognised to be a powerful means of disseminating improved communication skills between service users and health professionals, and encouraging both staff and service users to accept a much greater role for patients in becoming actively involved in treatment decisions and healthcare outcomes (Keech 2004; Wykurz & Kelly 2002). The expert patient initiative currently being implemented throughout the UK National Health Service incorporates a commitment for all health professionals to receive training in the expanded role and benefits of SMPs.

In theory, everyone benefits from the expert patient initiative. Through genuine partnership with health professionals as co-producers of healthcare, patients achieve better symptomatic control and are enabled to live more active, independent lives and benefit from a more democratic and user-oriented service provision. An anticipated reduction in the volume and cost of healthcare is a particularly attractive feature for government (Appleby, Harrison & Devlin 2003; Guevara *et al.* 2003; Kendall 2001; Lorig 2000; Richards 2004; Skelton 2001). Proponents of SMPs point to the significant benefits they have already been shown to deliver including improved control of symptoms, increased self-efficacy and independence, as well as reduced hospital visits and GP consultations (Department of Health 2001b; Guevara *et al.* 2003; Lorig 2000).

Concern has also been expressed about the motives which underlie the enthusiasm for shifting so much responsibility for healthcare from the statutory services to the individual user, and the future implications of such a move for patient entitlement to healthcare (Coveney & Bunton 2003; Fitzgerald 1994; Galvin 2002; Guevara *et al.* 2003; Lee-Trewick 2001; Lorig 2000; Misselbrook 2001; Richards 2004; Richards, Reid & Watt 2003; Salmon & Hall 2003; Skelton 2001). Laymen have always assumed a large responsibility for health (Hannay 1979). The extent of their involvement has increased over recent decades (Rogers, Hassell & Nikolaas 1999). Many patients may be willing and able to increase their involvement in managing health problems, especially when these are chronic and enduring, but some may not. In reality there are very finite limits to the extent to which people can prevent illness and control health, especially as they become older. However, the current emphasis on patients' self-management of illness is directly linked to the idea that they can and also should 'choose health' (Department of Health 2005; Donaldson 2003).

Thus, one way of reading the expert patient programme is as both a strategy for redrawing and contracting state responsibility for healthcare, and as an intensification of the 'coercive healthism' (Misselbrook 2001) and techniques of self-surveillance by which concepts of health and illness are deployed as instruments of social control (Armstrong 1995; Fitzgerald 1994; Galvin 2002; Zola 1975). The idea that patients can literally 'choose health' and that it is the role of government to facilitate such choices is a convenient propaganda (Department of Health 2003). Individualising illness in this way conveniently diverts attention from the structural determinants of health, and in particular the role of social and economic inequality and environmental factors as major causes of disease

(Jacobsen, Smith & Whitehead 1991; Townsend, Davidson & Whitehead 1990; Wilkinson 1996).

There is much to be gained from the development of genuine 'partnership' between patients and healthcare workers, and an increased awareness and understanding of the patient perspective by professionals. However, there are different ways in which these can be developed and it is not at all clear that the delegation of responsibility for illness and healthcare from the professional sector to the individual patient constitutes a particularly 'patient-centred' move, or that it corresponds to what patients themselves want from healthcare. 'Partnership', 'expert patient', 'patient-centred medicine', 'shared decision making' and even 'concordance' are professional, rather than lay, constructs. They represent professional or policy ideas and assumptions about how to improve services and deliver more efficient and cost-effective care and the kind of changes and services patients would like to experience. The extent of their relevance to patients has yet to be established. A growing body of evidence reveals patients' preferences for involvement in healthcare to be complex and often equivocal. In certain circumstances, where patients' sense of vulnerability and dependency prompts them to search for actively managed care, paternalism may be actively preferred (Lee-Trewick 2001; Lupton 1997; McKinstry & McKee 2000; Misselbrook 2001). To hand patients responsibility for healthcare without also providing access to the information and skills required to enable decision making and effective negotiation with health professionals is invidious. To impose the responsibility for self-management of illness on people who do not want it is as brutal and inappropriate as the denial of expertise and autonomy among those for whom active involvement in healthcare is a reflex coping mechanism. It is difficult to get the balance right.

The Expert Patient programme places great emphasis on the development of partnership between patients and professionals. It includes an obligation for professionals to *learn* about the experience of illness from patients who are co-opted as teachers within the medical curriculum. However, it is evident that the programme is oriented to a view of self-help which implies patient acceptance of conventional medical knowledge and expertise and a goal for patients to optimise the healthcare they receive from professionals, rather than engineer a radical change in health service culture. SMPs aim to provide patients with practical help and support to reduce their dependency on health service input. They also encourage patients to optimise the benefits of professional healthcare through cooperation and compliance with biomedical treatment and goals. SMPs may deliver substantial benefits for illness sufferers. However, they do not start with what patients want from the system, or the kind of system patients want, but rather train them to operate more effectively within the existing status quo. There is no recognition of the intrinsic conflicts between patients and professionals, or analysis of the frustrations and dissatisfactions experienced by all participants in the delivery and receipt of healthcare. There is a great difference between this concept of the expert or 'professional' patient and the original notion of the 'expert patient' put forward by Tuckett *et al.* (1985). This did not deny the gap in technical knowledge or expertise between patients and doctors, or necessarily seek to eliminate it. Patient expertise derived largely from *experience* and the individual's knowledge of his lived-in body. This was what the patient needed to be able to share with the doctor, and the doctor needed to be aware of. Patient expertise, in this view, is largely innate and experiential rather than something that has to be acquired through training and formal instruction. To a large extent, the Expert Patient initiative can be viewed as a further instance of incorporation rather than transformation as an adaptive strategy of an established professional practice confronted by pressure to change.

The user perspective

The view of the 'domesticated' or 'professional' patient within the Expert Patient programme is a far cry from the more radical conception of patient expertise which originated in the user movement of the 1960s to oppose the power and narrow professional focus of orthodox medicine (*see* Chapter 3). These empha-sised the *difference* between patients and professionals in their valuation of healthcare outcomes and treatment methods and goals, and the need for change in professional, far more than user, education and agendas (Rose 2001). In this view, self-help is motivated by *dissatisfaction* with service provision and *concern* about professional competence (Shapiro, Mosqueda & Botros 2003). Particularly in the field of mental health, such critical users felt they needed to acquire knowledge to compensate for the lack of understanding and therapeutic ineffectiveness of their doctors and to protect themselves from the harmful effects of what they experienced to be a damaging and abusive psychiatric system. Since the anti-psychiatry movement of the 1960s an extensive literature has docu-mented both continuing professional criticism and user dissatisfaction with psychiatric care, particularly the dominance of the biomedical model of mental illness and over-reliance on drugs as the major, and often only, treatment modality. The importance of patients having access to good quality information about their treatment, and complaints about widespread inadequacies of such provision are also recurrent themes throughout the literature (Arscott 1999; Barnes & Shardlow 1996; Boyle 1990; Bracken & Thomas 2001; Breggin 1993; Campbell 1996; Crossely 1998; Crossley & Crossley 2001; Depression Alliance 2002; Double 2002; Faulkener 1997; Ingleby 1981; Johnstone 2000; Kilian *et al.* 2003; Laing 1960; Laing & Esterson 1970; Newnes, Holmes & Dunn 1999; Newnes, Holmes & Dunn 2001; Perkins & Repper 1999; Read & Reynolds 1996; Rogers, Pilgrim & Lacey 1993; Rose 2001; Sainsbury Centre for Mental Health 1998; Szasz 1970; Szasz 1972; Treacher & Baruch 1981).

User organisations in the field of mental health tend to have a more radical political agenda than other voluntary organisations in campaigning for the extension and protection of citizenship rights for service users, as well as improvements in the quality of psychiatric provision and increased involvement of patients and carers in decisions about healthcare (Campbell 1996; Wallcroft & Bryant 2003). National user support organisations such as MIND and the National Schizophrenia Fellowship (now Rethink) have been influential in lobbying for improvements in the quality and user friendliness of services as well as the social profile of mental health and illness. Several effective user networks were formed in the mid-1980s to provide mutual support and have added weight to the campaign for change and resistance to the dominance of the formal psychiatric system: The UK Advocacy Network (UKAN), Survivors Speak Out, National Voices Network and The Hearing Voices Network (Wallcroft & Bryant 2003).

Although formally included within the mainstream policy and professional initiatives for patient-centred medicine (Department of Health 1999a, 2000, 2001c; NICE 2002; Royal College of Psychiatrists 2001), the status of mental health service users as expert patients is not clear (Richards 2004; Rose 2001). Recent documents and treatment guidelines contain exemplary statements about developing partnerships with mental health service users, tailoring services in accordance with user-defined needs and outcomes and involving patients in decisions about treatment (Department of Health 2001c; NICE 2002). For example, the government 'vision' of mental health services in the future includes a commitment to an 'equal partnership' between mental health service users and professionals, as well as users' entitlement to full citizenship along with the basic material needs required to support this (Department of Health 2001c). The first aim in the Mental Health Task Force mission statement is to 'treat individuals living with mental health problems with dignity and encourage their full involvement in their care' (Department of Health 2002b). Elsewhere, however, this message is muted or equivocal. The NHS Plan and the Expert Patient tend towards inclusiveness, but contain few references to categories of mental illness, though the self-management programme of the Manic Depression Fellowship does feature as an exemplar in the Expert Patient (Department of Health 2000, 2001b). The National Service Framework for Mental Health is another key document (Department of Health 1999a). Here, however, the position of mental health service users and the extent to which they can be acknowledged as potentially 'expert' appears much more uncertain. The involvement of service users in the development of their care plans is encouraged. This is recognised as being desirable both because users want it, and because the quality of care and associated outcomes improve when users are actively involved in managing their illness. However, when the context moves to consider medication, the frame of reference shifts back to 'compliance', and ways of ensuring that medicines are taken as prescribed. Indeed, 'compliance therapy' is advocated as a means of encouraging patients to accept treatment (Department of Health 1999a: 45, 46, 130). There is similar confusion and inconsistency in the NICE guidelines for treatment of schizophrenia (NICE 2002). Information should be provided, informed consent obtained, and service user preferences must be considered central to treatment decisions. However, there is no questioning of the *need* for antipsychotic medication, that adherence remains a clinical priority or that coercive treatments and involuntary detention may be necessary in some cases. User choice effectively comes down to selection of drug, rather than mode of treatment.

Beyond the gloss of rhetoric, there is little evidence that the policy goals relating to 'empowerment' of mental health service users, and their 'partnership' with professionals have made significant inroads into changing practice. Recent findings relating to user experiences of psychiatric hospitalisation and treatment continue to be largely critical and negative (Billcliff, McCabe & Brown 2001; Cobb, Darton & Kiran 2001; Corry, Hogman & Sandamas 2002; Department of Health 2001c; Kilian *et al.* 2003; Kmietowicz 2004; NICE 2002; Pollock *et al.* 2004; Quirk & Lelliott 2001; Rethink *et al.* 2004; Rose 2001; Sharkey 2002; Smith 2002a). It is hard to see how they could be otherwise while psychiatry retains the power to impose involuntary detention and coercive treatment: compulsion is not compatible with partnership. We could predict that if psychiatric services were becoming more patient-centred and user-friendly, compulsory detention of patients would be reduced. It is noteworthy, however, that this is reported to have increased by nearly 30% in the decade from 1992 to 2003 (Rethink *et al.* 2004). A substantial Sainsbury Centre survey found that although the majority (85%) of psychiatric hospital admissions were voluntary, an increasing number of patients were subject to a period of compulsory detention as their stay extended (Sainsbury Centre for Mental Health 1998). Running alongside the policy themes of patient partnership and inclusive citizenship is another, competing discourse about risk (Department of Health 1999a). Psychiatric patients, or at least a proportion of those who are most severely disturbed, are represented as posing a threat to social order. The containment of this threat justifies draconian measures including compulsory hospitalisation and medicine taking, and an emphasis on enforcing policies of compliance. The general tone of the NSF relating to mental health reinforces the privileged position of the dominant biomedical models of psychiatric practice. At the bottom line, professional judgement remains definitive and the legitimacy and also the difference of patient preferences for treatment and user-defined outcomes of care are unacknow-ledged and overwritten. 'Engaging' users in this context refers to engineering commitment and obedience among the minority of severely ill patients who are otherwise 'difficult' to contain cooperatively within the psychiatric system (Department of Health 1999a).

It appears that the notion of the 'expert patient' does not extend to users of mental health services. This group of particularly vulnerable people constitutes a test case for government policy and setting the limits of concordance. Precisely because the power differential between professionals and mental health service users is so great, it is more than usually necessary to advocate and protect patient preferences and values, and institute firm processes for eliciting, incorporating and respecting patient goals and choices for care and treatment. The prioritisation of patient experience over professional expertise is a longstanding feature of the user movement. Its internalisation within the mainstream health services would signal the start of a radical shift in the balance of power and a major reappraisal of the role of health professional (Bracken & Thomas 2001; Rogers, Pilgrim & Lacey 1993).

The internet

In recent years the internet has emerged as an unrivalled source of specialist knowledge for just about everything, especially health and disease. While concerns remain about the uneven distribution of access among different sectors of the population, internet use is spreading rapidly and is already established as a key resource for consumer information (Cotten & Gupta 2004; Coulter 2002b; Eysenbach & Jadad 2001; Garlick 2003; Gillespie, Florin & Gillam 2002; Hardey 1999; Jadad 1999). Garlic states that in two years between May 2000 and May 2002 the number of people accessing the internet in the UK had risen from approximately 19 million to 34 million: over half the population (Garlick 2003). Among those who use the internet, searching for health information is a very common practice. Jorgensen *et al.* state that an average of 23% of the EU population use the internet to find out about health issues. Denmark has the highest rate, at 47% of the population (Jorgensen & Gotzsche 2004). By 2004 more than 70 000 websites contained a focus on health with the number increasing rapidly (Cotten & Gupta 2004). The internet's immediate impact and future implications for the ways in which patients access healthcare and their relationships with professionals are not yet clear.

The internet is a resource of enormous potential in the dissemination of knowledge. In eroding the traditional medical monopoly of specialist information and blurring the boundary between lay and expert knowledge, it should be a powerful catalyst towards the development of the expert patient and the demo-cratisation of relationships between patients and healthcare professionals. Where knowledge is used as a strategy for coping with illness, the internet can serve as a positive resource for patients seeking to recover a sense of personal control and agency (Arnold 2003; Bentham 2004; Ziebland *et al.* 2004). There are concerns about the potentially divisive effects and increasing health inequalities among those who lack the resources or expertise to access the internet (Jadad 1999; Rozmovits & Ziebland 2004; Ziebland *et al.* 2004). Alongside these, however, it can enable people who would not otherwise have engaged with formal healthcare to access information and advice. The anonymity of the internet encourages the search for information about sensitive or personal topics that patients can be reluctant to discuss with their doctors (Cohen *et al.* 2001; Ziebland *et al.* 2004).

Ziebland *et al.* investigated the ways in which cancer patients used the internet as a resource in checking and interpreting information, seeking further opinions, sharing experiences and getting support from other sufferers (Ziebland *et al.* 2004). They concluded that the internet was meeting needs that were unlikely to be provided by other means, including the professional health services. In particular, they suggest that mastering the technology of the internet, and gaining knowledge and expertise in relation to their disease, provides patients with a way of asserting a kind of personal competence which helps them to resist the loss of self-esteem and social value which often follows serious illness.

Dynamic and interactive media such as online chat rooms, helplines and discussion forums provide patients with access to social support as well as information within world wide virtual communities. Sharing the *experience* of other sufferers, and the expertise which is born from this, is highly valued by many patients (Hardey 2002; Rozmovits & Ziebland 2004). Hardey highlights the significance of personal web authorship, and the sharing of personal experience with others.

> Within newsgroups, chatrooms and other interactive resources people 'open up' to others in an environment where anonymity promotes trust in strangers. Such electronic communities offer new opportun-ities for people with chronic or debilitating conditions to participate on an equal basis in community life. Global self-help groups provide a space for strangers who are bound within an environment that minimises the 'gamble' (Giddens 1991) involved in sharing intimate feelings.
>
> Hardey (1999: 831)*

The internet provides access to a range and diversity of information and experience which individual users must sift and appraise for themselves. This

---

* Hardey (1999) Reproduced with permission from Blackwell Publishing, Oxford.

in itself provides a stimulus for critical reflection and demystification of the expert knowledge supplied by health professionals. The particular salience of *experiential* rather than theoretical knowledge among web authors prioritises a new kind of expertise. This presents a challenge to the traditional authority of professionals with the potential to realign their relationships with patients (Hardey 1999). Cohen *et al.* further comment on the way in which the internet is dissolving the boundaries between lay and expert knowledge, as laymen become not only expert patients, but also *producers* rather than merely consumers of information (Cohen *et al.* 2001). They point to the potential value of patients' expertise in advancing professional knowledge and practice, especially in relation to the reporting of the adverse effects of new drugs. For example, patients were using the internet to air concerns about the problems associated with antidepressants, including addiction and dependency, long before these were formally recognised and acted on by professionals and official agencies (Cohen *et al.* 2001; Medawar *et al.* 2002).

In providing information which enables people to decide when it is necessary to seek medical help, the internet could result in a reduced demand on services, or at least promote their more effective and appropriate use (Coulter 2002b). Bentham describes the case of a mother who used the internet to accurately diagnose her child as suffering from diabetes. In taking this initiative, which included using diagnostic urine markers purchased from a pharmacist, the mother streamlined the process of diagnosis and referral and incurred personal costs, in both time and money, with a consequent saving on NHS resources. This example provides a good illustration of the expert patient in action, and points to ways in which government objectives to switch costs and responsibility from the public to the private sector could be advanced. Additional measures include the direct delivery of health interventions such as cognitive behaviour therapy (Christensen, Griffiths & Jorm 2004) and supplementing the time and resources patients can receive directly from clinicians through providing downloadable information materials including treatment decision aids as well as online access to professionals by email and videoconferencing (Street 2003).

Given its challenge to established conventions of medical practice and authority, it is not surprising that the professional response to the internet as a resource for patients has been generally negative if not dismissive (Eysenbach & Jadad 2001; Malone *et al.* 2004; Rozmovits & Ziebland 2004; Ziebland *et al.* 2004). Professional resistance tends to be voiced in terms of concern about the variable quality of online material. Since patients are assumed to lack the competence and critical appraisal skills to discriminate between accurate and misleading information, they are thought likely to be misled – perhaps even exploited and harmed – by material they access on the internet (Coleman 2003; Jorgensen & Gotzsche 2004). However, there is evidence to suggest that many people are already aware of the pitfalls of the internet, and tend to be quite cautious and critical in their use of it (Coleman 2003; Hardey 1999; Rozmovits & Ziebland 2004), though this is not always the case (Henwood *et al.* 2003). Rozmovits and Ziebland found that respondents often validated information by comparing several different sources (Rozmovits & Ziebland 2004). The internet might prove to be an effective stimulus for a more general critical evaluation of health information, which may then be turned back to appraise material accessed through formal health services and professionals (Hardey 1999; Hardey 2002). The development of various tools and checklists to increase consumer competence, along with the kite marking of 'quality approved' sites to help this process is already underway (Briscoe 2003; Charnock 1998; Kiley & Graham 2002; Rees, Ford & Sheard 2002; Wilson 2002).

Studies directly evaluating the quality of health information on patient websites have returned mixed findings. Sandvik concluded that the internet was an excellent source of mainly accurate information about urinary incontinence, and that interactive email and chat services provided valuable comfort and advice to users (Sandvik 1999). Jorgensen and Gotzsche (2004) found that three (financially) independent consumer groups provided the best information about mammographic screening for women (Jorgensen & Gotzsche 2004). Thirteen sites from industry sponsored advocacy groups and 11 sites produced by government institutions all presented partial and highly selective information which was strongly biased in favour of screening. The authors concluded that these sites would not have enabled women to assess the benefits and harms or make a properly informed decision of mammography. Although consumers tend to be wary of commercial sites, embedded sponsorship is often hard to spot. Herxheimer has commented on the problem of bias introduced into the websites of voluntary patient support organisations who come to depend on the financial sponsorship of pharmaceutical companies (Herxheimer 2003). For less obvious reasons, the quality of web information attributed directly to doctors has also been found inaccurate or misleading (McPherson 1999).

Alongside genuine concerns about the quality of internet content, professional resistance also derives from the threat posed by patient expertise. This insecurity is expressed in the ubiquitous negative stereotype of the demanding patient who attends the consultation equipped with his internet printout of inappropriate or inaccurate information. The stereotype persists despite empirical findings that patients are rarely prepared to disclose internet information in the consultation (Cotten & Gupta 2004; Henwood *et al.* 2003; Kohner & Hill 2000; Malone *et al.* 2004). Malone *et al.* found that GPs regarded patients who presented downloaded information in the consultation as 'demanding', and adopted strategies to contain or discourage such challenges. The doctors in their study also differentiated patient approaches according to context. They recognised the legitimacy of patients seeking further information about controversial issues such as the MMR vaccine, and they approved of patients with an established diagnosis who used the internet to gain supplementary information about their illness and how to manage it. However, they disapproved of patients who attempted to self-diagnose or identify appropriate treatments prior to the consultation and so presumably arrived with pre-formed theories about the nature of the problem and what should be done about it (Malone *et al.* 2004).

Some clinicians have recognised the usefulness of the internet as a source of information for patients and its potential to improve both medical care and relationships (Arnold 2003; Bentham 2004; Goldsmith 1999; Josh 2003; Street 2003). An inspirational account of how effectively the internet may be used as a resource to benefit both patients and doctors, and how a problem might be transformed into an opportunity is given in a letter to the BMJ by John Goldsmith which is reproduced in Box 8.1 (Goldsmith 1999). In this view of the future, the doctor will no longer be the only or even the main source of information about health and illness. Patients will increasingly access knowledge from a wide range of media outside the medical consultation and bring the results of their reflection and research to discuss with their doctors and other health professionals. Coulter suggests that there may be a new role for designated 'information brokers' working in different healthcare settings. Where, as is often the case, patients require only information and reassurance, the broker could deal with many enquiries pre-emptively, avoiding further consultations with more specialist clinical staff (Coulter 2002b).

Box 8.1 Patients and families as partners – sharing the burden of knowledge

Sir, Many families attend my clinics with problems which defy the text-books or for which there is little useful information available in the usual sources (public library etc.). Examples include syndromic disorders (chromosomal and non-chromosomal), pervasive developmental disorders such as autism, and unusual neurological, cardiac, dermatological and nutritional problems. Though individually rare, these can make up a significant portion of the total workload of the average paediatrician. Since the introduction of the internet, especially the Web, information on these conditions is now readily available to many families either from their own computer or through contact with one of the many support groups. These families often find information which is of uncertain quality or usefulness, and they are also prone to dismiss their researches when discussing their concerns in the context of a busy clinic.

Recently I have taken a greater interest in the information some families have found, and have actively engaged their own interest in finding useful material and helped them with useful starting points for their internet travels. To my surprise they are now often well-informed, much more up-to-date than I am able to be, and with support they can assume much of the responsibility for becoming 'experts' in their child's or family's condition. Indeed I now find that a peculiar feeling of relief has entered the consultation process, which in retrospect is one of 'sharing the burden of knowledge' with the family. No longer am I the source of all knowledge and the 'superior know-it-all'.

As a consequence, children and families which were previously regarded as difficult and time-consuming have become partners in an exciting adventure, with co-responsibility for deciding which steps to take next in the search for difficult answers about treatments and investigations, based on good information.

The effects on our 'doctor–patient' relationships have been difficult to quantify, but I feel certain that for many families, being given permission to be knowledgeable about their own problem has been therapeutic in its own right, and has been immensely useful as a source of clinically valuable information, provided the family accepts that some of what they find will be quackery.

John Goldsmith (1999)*

---

* John Goldsmith (1999) *BMJ*. **318**(19 March): eletters (bmj.bmjjournals.com/cgi/eletters/ 318/7186/DC1). Reproduced with permission from the BMJ Publishing Group.

Despite uneven public access, the internet has already had a very substantial impact as an information resource, and its potential to alter healthcare delivery in future is enormous. However, at the present time it is easy to overestimate its effects, and the extent to which independent information seeking is generalised throughout the population. For many patients, professionals remain the main, or only, source of information about illness (Cotten & Gupta 2004; Kirk, Kirk & Kristjanson 2004; Makoul, Arntson & Schofield 1995). This was the case for all but one of the 32 respondents in Henwood *et al.*'s study, only half of whom had ever used the internet to search for information about health (Henwood, Wyatt, Hart & Smith 2003). A significant minority did not regard it as necessary or appropriate to acquire knowledge independently, or to assume the responsibility for becoming actively involved in medical decision making. These studies also indicate that the internet is only one of a range of different media used to gain information, and that for many people, personal contacts such as family and friends remain much more important sources of advice and knowledge about matters relating to health (Budtz & Witt 2002).

Using knowledge

Regardless of whether patients get their expert information from the internet or somewhere else, there is considerable evidence to suggest that the tension between *having* knowledge, and feeling able, or entitled, to *display* it in the consultation remains unresolved (Heritage 1997). Many professionals feel challenged by the notion of the expert patient, while many patients still feel uncomfortable revealing their knowledge to professionals (Cotten & Gupta 2004; Henwood *et al.* 2003). Indeed, this etiquette is so strong that health professionals themselves have been observed to suspend their medical expertise and act like 'normal' patients when seeking medical help on their own behalf (Jaye & Wilson 2003; Strong 1979). In a personal account of his hospitalisation and surgery for cancer, Frank Arnold describes how he turned immediately to search the internet for detailed information about his condition and prognosis. He comments:

> I could have asked my consultant some of these questions but did not want to imply criticism of the excellent surgery and outcome.
>
> Arnold (2003: 1042)*

This extract illustrates the tension between being a 'good' patient and being an informed or enquiring one. Some of Leydon *et al.*'s respondents indicated that their reluctance to question staff or seek additional information stemmed not only from a sense that this was inappropriate, but that do to so indicated a lack of trust in their doctors (Leydon *et al.* 2000). The desire to present oneself as a good patient and the fear of alienating staff is a recurring theme throughout the literature. It testifies to the strength of patients' feelings of dependency and pressure to conform, especially among those who are more seriously ill (Burkitt Wright, Holcombe & Salmon 2004; Leydon *et al.* 2000; Radley 1996). In critical situations especially, patients manifest a need to *trust* in medical expertise and to

* Arnold F (2003) Reproduced with permission from the BMJ Publishing Group.

maintain hope: the quest for information is often a lesser priority. In a study of patients receiving palliative care for cancer respondents sometimes 'verbalised ambiguity': they wanted to be told but not to know. Even in the final stages of their illness, it was important for respondents to be able to maintain hope, and consequently for information to be tempered (Kirk, Kirk & Kristjanson 2004; Leydon *et al.* 2000).

In certain contexts, resisting information may be a preferred strategy for coping with the threat of illness. Radley observed how men undergoing heart surgery coped with their anxiety about the operation. Acceptance of the need for surgery was justified with reference to the expert judgement of clinicians who 'knew best'. Placing trust in the skills and ability of their surgeons removed the burden of responsibility from patients, and enabled them to feel secure about their outcome and prognosis. At this point respondents did not *want* more information which could have compromised their confidence. During follow-up interviews, however, once patients felt themselves to be back on firmer ground, Radley noticed that his respondents started to reappraise their need for information prior to the operation, and to indicate that they should have been better informed. In hindsight, and once the operation was safely over and recovery well advanced, they could allow themselves the indulgence of taking up a position which was closer to the autonomous consumer than the dependent patient they had once been (Radley 1996).

Radley's study shows how people's representations of their information needs may change with time and experience, as they continually rework and update the narrative of their illness. It also raises questions about how much information patients actually want, and how this can be assessed and tailored at any given time. We might ask, also, what it means when people say that they want to be 'fully informed' or to 'know everything'? Clearly, the latter is impossible, but perhaps there is a point at which people come to feel they know 'enough' – and this will vary very widely between different individuals, for different illnesses, and at different times. The proponents of comprehensive information provision tend to overlook the double edge of knowledge: its capacity to intensify fear and uncertainty just as it can also inspire confidence and a sense of control (Edwards, Elwyn & Mulley 2002). Leydon observed that some cancer patients found even basic information leaflets about their illness frightening (Leydon *et al.* 2000). Once revealed, information cannot be retracted or 'un-known' and people cannot anticipate in advance what they are going to find out, or what effects it will have on them. Seeking information involves a gamble, with the risks increasing in proportion to the severity of illness and threat to health. This may help to account for different findings about patients' preferences for health information, and the tendency for the active search for information to diminish with the urgency or seriousness of their condition (Burkitt Wright, Holcombe & Salmon 2004; Kirk, Kirk & Kristjanson 2004; Leydon *et al.* 2000).

Research methodology and context are important determinants of study outcomes. It makes a lot of difference whether people are well or ill, considering actual or hypothetical situations, and current, future or past events when they are asked about their desire for illness information. In contrast to the more guarded response of patients asked about their preferences when they were seriously ill, Berry *et al.* found that almost all (98%) of the healthy respondents presented with a set of hypothetical scenarios said they would prefer being given information about their condition to not (Berry, Gillie & Banbury 1995). A further complication is that people may be responding in terms that they feel are appropriate – providing a socially sanctioned 'public' rather than a personal 'private' account of what they think (Cornwell 1985).

Regardless of people's actual preferences, in the information age the patient role is changing. Ziebland *et al.* suggest that acquiring knowledge and a mastery of information technology constitute a kind of competence for cancer patients which helps to offset the socially diminishing and exclusionary aspects of their illness (Ziebland *et al.* 2004). More generally, in the government's vision of the 'expert patient' information is a prerequisite for assuming responsibility for health (Department of Health 2001b, 2003). It is not yet clear to what extent this model of the informed and autonomous consumer of healthcare more closely reflects patient preferences, or political and professional agendas and (albeit well intentioned) ideologies.

A situation where people feel obliged to conceal their knowledge or concerns in the interests of convention and the fear of alienating doctors is very far from satisfactory. West described the increasing alienation experienced by parents as they became more knowledgeable and confident in dealing with their child's epilepsy, but continued to be given little information by their doctors and excluded from involvement in discussion about treatment (West 1976). It is likely that in future, the frustration and resentment experienced by well informed patients who feel unable to present their knowledge and related questions for discussion will result in their increasing independence from, and consequent marginalisation of, professional health workers.

It is important that patients can access a wide range of high quality information about all aspects of their health and illness as a matter of routine. However, it is not the case that all patients want to do this, or that the effects of information are always benign. To make things more difficult, individual information needs are liable to change over time, and in different contexts. People may not know either the full extent of what *could* be known, or the questions for which they need answers. They may only find out what they need to know after the event, in reappraising and reconstructing the past. The preceding discussion has illustrated that the provision of information to patients is far from straightforward, and much more variable and uncertain than is usually assumed in current policy documents and the research literature. The current drive to manufacture 'expert patients' remains largely directed to meeting goals of the policy and professional agenda (increasing compliance and reducing cost) rather than directly addressing patient defined needs. Unwelcome side effects are manifesting themselves in patients' sense of *obligation* to acquire expertise in illness and an increase in the self-attribution of *blame* or failure for loss of health (Bissell, May & Noyce 2004; Johnson 1991; Lee-Trewick 2001; Moore, Chamberlain & Khuri 2004; Richards, Reid & Watt 2003).

The trend to involve patients in the development and evaluation of information materials is to be welcomed and should continue to be extended. Information materials that are constructed in collaboration with patients have been shown to differ in content and form from those devised solely by professionals (Jones *et al.* 2000; Kennedy, Robinson & Rogers 2003; Moumjid *et al.* 2003; Nair *et al.* 2002). Patients often prioritise different kinds of information from professionals and put knowledge to different uses. The clinical perspective is oriented to the elimination of symptoms and control of disease. Patients tend to privilege the *experience* of illness and treatment, and focus on strategies to protect normal routines and social obligations and maintain quality of life. In particular, they are concerned with the attribution of *meaning* to the arbitrary, chaotic and inexplicable experience of illness (Frank 1995; Hyden 1997; Kangas 2001; Kleinman 1988; Launer 2002; Williams 1984). Information is transmuted into knowledge as it filters through the prism of personal understanding, feelings, aspirations and experience. Individuals respond differently to the same information. This is why the goals of professional education programmes are so often subverted. Dixon-Woods has taken issue with the poverty of the 'mathematical model' of information transfer employed in the patient education discourse (Dixon-Woods 2001). From this perspective, education amounts to the transfer of a quantity of information from one source (professional) to another (patient), as if there was only one set of meanings to be derived from such transactions. The state of being adequately informed should automatically overwrite the misconceptions and inaccuracies which impede compliance. Remedying the information deficit should cause patients to understand the irrationality of failing to comply with medical advice and modify their behaviour accordingly (Horne & Weinman 2004).

A preoccupation with the layout, presentation and design of information materials, including the anticipated reading age of patients, stems from the assumption that the task of educating patients can be reduced to solving the technical problems of design and access. This overlooks that information is only turned into knowledge and understanding through the critical assessment and active construction of meaning by the recipient: 'it is readers, and not texts, who create meaning' (Dixon-Woods 2001: 1431). From the patient's perspective, information serves many purposes, and increasing compliance is not usually one of them. Simply providing patients with information will not automatically lead to improved communication or satisfaction. Knowing more may increase, rather than diminish, dissatisfaction, just as it may increase, rather than decrease, non-compliance. Further research is required to establish how people assess the credibility of different sources of knowledge, their preferences for mode of information delivery and how they respond to inconsistent and contradictory information from different sources. The existing literature suggests that many patients value verbal rather than written information, and the opportunities this offers for building relationships with professionals. The courtesy of taking time to talk to patients was valued for its demonstration of respect for the patient's autonomy and personal competence. However, patient disappointment with their experience of communication with professionals is widespread. It may be that when people report dissatisfaction with the information they have been given about their illness, they are primarily expressing dissatisfaction with their relationships with staff.

The evidence reviewed in the preceding discussion suggests that many patients may still consider deference to professional expertise to be appropriate and desirable. They may resist the attribution of greater personal responsibility for medical decision making that is assumed within the role of expert patient. However, patients desiring a more active role in the consultation are likely to experience frustration at being unable to share their knowledge with professionals, and even the sense of obligation to conceal what they know. Even expert patients can find it difficult to express their views and display their knowledge.

Formal deference to professional expertise and the idealisation of professional knowledge and patient ignorance effectively disables the patient contribution. Good information without the scope or opportunity for good communication will produce patients who are disaffected and alienated from the formal healthcare system (West 1976).

Professional hierarchy and organisational complexity

The patient education discourse operates with an idealised view of encounters between patients and professionals. These are portrayed as taking place between autonomous individuals in some kind of clear white space, untrammelled by constraints of context or organizational setting. The patient–professional dyad is considered in isolation from the complex interprofessional and interpersonal relationships that anchor individuals within complex networks of obligation, allegiance and exchange. In a study of treatment information provision to patients on acute psychiatric wards, Pollock *et al.* identified features of professional hierarchy and organisational complexity which restricted patients' access to information (Pollock, Grime, Baker & Mantala 2004). Staff and patients agreed that the current provision of information was unsatisfactory. Patients were not provided with specific information about medicines unless they made a point of asking, which most did not. Staff also broadly supported patients' entitlement to information and the commitment to greater patient involvement in healthcare. However, particularly among the hospital-based clinical staff, and especially the nurses, there was considerable ambivalence about providing patients with information. Parsimonious disclosure was used more or less deliberately as a strategy of patient management. The professional hierarchy also blocked transmission of information to patients as staff were wary of transgressing interdisciplinary boundaries. Junior staff, in particular, felt constrained by the disclosure practices of more senior colleagues, particularly the consultants, which they felt the need to uphold. Similar findings were reported by Stapleton, Kirkham & Thomas in a study of information provision in the very different setting of antenatal clinics (Stapleton, Kirkham & Thomas 2002). This suggests that the professional hierarchy works to obstruct the realisation of concordance across a range of healthcare settings, not just mental health.

Other studies have described the adverse effects for patients of interprofessional deference and tension (Hughes & McCann 2003). Pharmacists show reluctance to address patient concerns about medicines directly, for fear of appearing to challenge the doctors' authority and clinical judgement (Lambert 1995; Reebye *et al.* 2002). Patients raising questions or seeking advice are likely to be referred back to the GP, or other professional, who may well be the source of their concern. This is not only onerous, but also a difficult and unwelcome task to hand the patient (Landers 2002), who ends up being an intermediary absorbing the inconsistencies between different professionals and agencies. This is likely to become more of an issue with the extension of supplementary prescribing. The tightly circumscribed and delegated authority of nurse and pharmacist prescribers effectively minimises their scope for autonomous decision making and constrains the candour of their discussions with patients (Dowell 2004). These findings demonstrate the necessity of extending the analysis of concordance to take account of the extent to which communication in medical consultations is moulded by the wider networks of professional relationships and organisational structures extending far beyond the simple patient-professional dyad.

Given the difficulty of realising concordance in single consultations, the prospect of achieving and extending shared understandings throughout a complex chain of encounters involving a multiplicity of staff from different professional specialities is more than daunting. In a study of how users of mental health services cope with complexity in the provision of healthcare, respondents reported problems with accessing services, establishing good relationships with professionals and maintaining continuity of relationships to be greater concerns than the provision of specific information about medicines (Pollock & Grime 2004). Most service users in the study tended to assume they lacked the necessary expertise to get involved in treatment decisions, and regarded these as more appropriately matters of professional judgement. Respondents expressed awareness of the professional hierarchy – with themselves at the bottom – and its impact on their experience and evaluation of care. For example, some considered that their GPs lacked the necessary expertise to deal with serious mental illness and did not expect them to have any further involvement following specialist referral. Others valued a more holistic approach to care. Some people felt their GPs no longer wanted to deal with problems for which they were receiving specialist attention, and took referral as an opportunity for disengagement from involvement in these. In the case of complex health problems involving referrals to several specialist agencies this could lead to a very fragmented experience of care. This study also found that non-prescribing professionals were reluctant to step beyond the boundaries of their role and were rarely prepared to discuss medicines directly with patients. Interprofessional deference helps to reduce tension and conflict within the workforce but contributes to a fragmentation of care for patients. Commitment to the maintenance of a consistent professional front precludes the open discussion of many patient concerns. Professionals were rarely prepared to express disagreement or direct criticisms of other health workers. This prioritising of corporate interests can make it very difficult for patients to discuss many of their concerns directly with professionals. It results in a form of censorship in communication with patients which works directly against the achievement of concordance.

Respondents seemed routinely to be passive recipients of services and treatments. Medicines were prescribed and referrals made with little or no explanation of their purpose, duration and expected outcome. Individual staff and services came and went in an unpredictable and arbitrary fashion. Respondents seemed largely passive and powerless to influence the direction and quality of care, or to achieve the personalisation of a service tailored to their individual preferences and needs. Service provision remained based on professional assessment of user needs and professional evaluation of the therapeutic gain from service input. The process of referral was often experienced as arbitrary and impersonal. In particular, users had little ability to influence the duration and continuation of services, such as counselling, that they regarded as beneficial.

These studies indicate that it is not so much having information about the technicalities of treatment that determines whether patients can play an active part in decisions about care, but ignorance of their case and the inability to influence the disposal of resources. The kind of knowledge users need, but often cannot access, concerns the nature, availability and entitlement to services, as well as information and understanding about the *process* of care: what decisions have been made about them, by whom, and what are the implications and consequences that flow from these (Rose 2001)? For mental health service users in particular, nothing is more disempowering than the inability to access, modify or certify the medical record that others have compiled about them. Transparency of information at this level is required if patients are to be involved in healthcare in any meaningful way, and to achieve genuine inclusion as members of the therapeutic 'team' (Sang 2004). Coulter regards it as extraordinary that patients' access to their medical records has been withheld until relatively recently (Coulter 2002b). It is still very far from routine. The requirement (since April 2004) of copying patients in on correspondence between the professionals involved in their case is a very welcome development (Smith 2002b). It remains to be seen how patients respond, and in what ways it might influence the forms of communication between professionals and with patients.

Conclusion

The commitment to patient information among professionals and policy makers has become almost a reflex response. Patient entitlement and easy access to as much high quality information as they desire is uncontestable. However, the evidence reviewed in the preceding discussion points to the need to rethink the role and purpose of patient information, and to expand the focus from treatment options to the wider processes of case management and resource allocation. In particular, questions have been raised about the nature and extent of patient demand for information, and how this varies between individuals and different healthcare settings. The tension between the desire for trust and dependency and informed autonomy needs much further investigation, and so does the experience of knowledge as a threat or burden, rather than a positive resource. The impact of modern information technologies in redefining the competence of individual citizens is not yet clear, nor is the patient response to expansion of the sick role to incorporate a much greater personal responsibility for health. It is evident, however, that concordance should not be confused with techniques of providing information to patients, or reduced to a covert strategy to increase compliance.

References

Appleby J, Harrison A and Devlin N (2003) *What is the Real Cost of More Patient Choice?* King's Fund, London.

Armstrong D (1995) The rise of surveillance medicine. *Sociology of Health and Illness.* **17**(3): 393–404.

Arnold F (2003) Patient power? *BMJ.* **326**(10 May): 1042.

Arscott KJ (1999) ECT: The facts psychiatry declines to mention. In: C Newnes, G Holmes and C Dunn (eds) *This is Madness: a critical look at psychiatry and the future of mental health services.* PCCS Books, Ross-on-Wye, pp. 95–113.

Asscher AW, Parr GD and Whitmarsh VB (1995) Towards the safer use of medicines. *BMJ.* **311**(14 October): 1003–5.

Barnes M and Shardlow P (1996) Identity Crisis: Mental health user groups and the 'problem' of identity. In: C Barnes and G Mercer (eds) *Exploring the Divide.* The Disability Press, Leeds, pp. 114–34.

Beach WA, Easter DW, Good JS and Pigeron E (2005) Disclosing and responding to cancer 'fears' during oncology interviews. *Social Science and Medicine.* **60**: 893–910.

Beck U (1992) *Risk Society: towards a new modernity.* Sage Publications, London.

Bellaby P (2001) Evidence and risk: the sociology of health care grappling with knowledge and uncertainty. In: A Edwards and G Elwyn (eds) *Evidence-based Patient Choice: inevitable or impossible?* Oxford University Press, Oxford, pp. 78–94.

Bentham J (2004) The internet – friend or foe? *BMJ.* **328**(17 January): 133.

Berry DC, Gillie T and Banbury S (1995) What do patients want to know: an empirical approach to explanation generation and validation. *Expert Systems With Applications.* **8**(4): 419–28.

Billcliff N, McCabe E and Brown KW (2001) Informed consent to medication in long-term psychiatric in-patients. *Psychiatric Bulletin.* **25**: 132–4.

Bissell P, May C and Noyce PR (2004) From compliance to concordance: barriers to accomplishing a re-framed model of health care interactions. *Social Science and Medicine.* **58**: 851–62.

Boyle M (1990) *Schizophrenia: a scientific delusion?* Routledge, London.

Bracken P and Thomas P (2001) Postpsychiatry: a new direction for mental health. *BMJ.* **322**(24 March): 724–7.

Breggin P (1993) *Toxic Psychiatry, Drugs and Electroconvulsive Therapy: the truth and better alternatives.* HarperCollins, London.

Briscoe M (2003) *Webguide: evaluating the quality of health information on the Internet.* Royal College of Psychiatrists. www.rcpsych.ac.uk/info/webguide/quality.htm

Budtz S and Witt K (2002) Consulting the Internet before visit to general practice: patients' use of the Internet and other sources of health information. *Scandanavian Journal of Primary Health Care.* **20**: 174–6.

Burkitt Wright E, Holcombe C and Salmon P (2004) Doctors' communication of trust, care, and respect in breast cancer: qualitative study. *BMJ.* **328**(10 April): 864–7.

Campbell P (1996) The history of the user movement in the United Kingdom. In: T Heller *et al.* (eds) *Mental Health Matters, A Reader.* Macmillan/Open University, London, pp. 218–26.

Campbell P, Cobb A and Darton K (1998) *Psychiatric Drugs: users' experiences and current policy and practice.* Mind Publications, London.

Chaplin R and Kent A (1998) Informing patients about tardive dyskinesia. Controlled trial of patient education. *British Journal of Psychiatry.* **172**: 78–81.

Charnock D (1998) *The DISCERN Handbook: quality criteria for consumer health information on treatment choices.* Radcliffe Medical Press, Oxford.

Christensen H, Griffiths K and Jorm AF (2004) Delivering interventions for depression by using the internet: randomised controlled trial. *BMJ.* **328**: 265.

Cobb A, Darton K and Kiran J (2001) *Mind's Yellow Card for Reporting Drug Side Effects: a report of users' experiences.* Mind Publications, London.

Cohen D, McCubbin M, Collin J and Perodeau G (2001) Medications as social phenomena. *Health.* **5**(4): 441–69.

Cohen H and Britten N (2003) Who decides about prostate cancer treatment? A qualitative study. *Family Practice.* **20**(6): 724–9.

Coleman B (2003) Producing an information leaflet to help patients access high quality drug information on the Internet: a local study. *Health Information and Libraries Journal.* **20**: 160–71.

Cornwell J (1985) *Hard Earned Lives: accounts of health and illness from East London.* Tavistock, London.

Corrigan O (2003) Empty ethics: the problem with informed consent. *Sociology of Health and Illness.* **25**(3): 768–92.

Corry P, Hogman G and Sandamas G (2002) *That's Just Typical.* NSF, London.

Cotten SR and Gupta SS (2004) Characteristics of online and offline health information seekers and factors that discriminate between them. *Social Science and Medicine.* **59**(9): 1795–806.

Coulter A (2002a), After Bristol: putting patients at the centre. *BMJ*. **324**(16 March): 648–51.

Coulter A (2002b) *The Autonomous Patient: ending paternalism in medical care*. The Nuffield Trust, London.

Coulter A, Entwistle V and Gilbert D (1998) *Informing Patients: an assessment of the quality of patient information materials*. King's Fund, London.

Coulter A, Entwistle V and Gilbert D (1999) Sharing decisions with patients: is the information good enough? *BMJ*. **318**: 318–22.

Coveney J and Bunton R (2003) In pursuit of the study of pleasure: implications for health research and practice. *Health*. **7**(2): 161–79.

Crawford MJ and Kessel AS (1999) Not listening to patients – the use and misuse of patient satisfaction studies. *International Journal of Social Psychiatry*. **45**(1): 1–7.

Crawford R (1977) You are dangerous to your health: the ideology and politics of victim blaming. *International Journal of Health Services*. **7**: 663–80.

Crawford R (2004) Risk ritual and the management of control and anxiety in medical culture. *Health*. **8**(4): 505–28.

Crossely N (1998) RD Laing and the British anti-psychiatry movement: a socio-historical analysis. *Social Science and Medicine*. **47**(7): 877–89.

Crossley ML and Crossley N (2001) 'Patient' voices, social movements and the habitus; how psychiatric survivors 'speak out'. *Social Science and Medicine*. **52**(10): 1377–94.

Department of Health (1991) *The Patient's Charter*. Department of Health, London.

Department of Health (1996) *Patient Partnership: building a collaborative strategy*. Department of Health, National Health Service Executive, London.

Department of Health (1998) *Our Healthier Nation: a contract for health*. Department of Health, London.

Department of Health (1999a) *A National Service Framework for Mental Health*. Department of Health, London.

Department of Health (1999b) *Patient and Public Involvement in the New NHS*. Department of Health, London.

Department of Health (2000) *The NHS Plan: a plan for investment, a plan for reform*. Department of Health, London.

Department of Health (2001a) *Good Practice in Consent Implementation Guide: consent to examination or treatment*. Department of Health, London.

Department of Health (2001b) *The Expert Patient: a new approach to chronic disease management for the 21st Century*. Department of Health, London.

Department of Health (2001c) *The Journey to Recovery: the government's vision for mental health care*. Department of Health, London.

Department of Health (2002a) *Learning from Bristol: the DH response to the report of the public inquiry into children's heart surgery at the Bristol Royal Infirmary 1984–1995*. Department of Health, London.

Department of Health (2002b) *Mental Health Task Force: an introduction*. Department of Health, London.

Department of Health (2003) *Building on the Best, Choice, Responsiveness and Equity in the NHS*. Department of Health, London.

Department of Health (2005) *Delivering Choosing Health: making healthier choices easier*. Department of Health, London.

Depression Alliance (2002) *Depression and Antidepressants*. Depression Alliance, London.

Dickinson D, Raynor DK and Duman M (2001) Patient information leaflets for medicines: using consumer testing to determine the most effective design. *Patient Education and Counselling*. **43**(2): 147–59.

Dixon-Woods M (2001) Writing wrongs? An analysis of published discourses about the use of patient information leaflets. *Social Science and Medicine*. **52**(9): 1417–32.

Donaldson L (2003) Expert patients usher in a new era of opportunity for the NHS. *BMJ*. **326**(14 June): 1279–80.

Double D (2002) The limits of psychiatry. *BMJ.* **324**: 900–4.

Dowell J (2004) The prescriber's perspective. In: C Bond (ed.) *Concordance: a partnership in medicine taking.* Pharmaceutical Press, London, pp. 49–70.

Edwards A and Elwyn G (2001) *Evidence-based Patient Choice: inevitable or impossible?* Oxford University Press, Oxford.

Edwards A, Elwyn G and Mulley A (2002) Explaining risks: turning numerical data into meaningful pictures. *BMJ.* **324**: 827–30.

Elwyn G, Edwards A, Gwyn R and Grol R (1999a) Towards a feasible model for shared decision making: focus group study with general practitioners. *BMJ.* **319**: 753–6.

Elwyn G, Gwyn R, Edwards A and Grol R (1999b) Is 'shared decision making' feasible in consultations for upper respiratory tract infections? Assessing the influence of antibiotic expectations using discourse analysis. *Health Expectations.* **2**: 105–17.

Eysenbach G and Jadad AR (2001) Consumer health informatics in the Internet age. In: A Edwards and G Elwyn (eds) *Evidence-Based Patient Choice: Inevitable or Impossible?* Oxford University Press, Oxford, pp. 289–307.

Faulkener A (1997) *Knowing Our Own Minds: a survey of how people in emotional distress take control of their lives.* Mental Health Foundation, London.

Faulkener A and Thomas P (2002) User-led research and evidence-based medicine. *British Journal of Psychiatry.* **180**: 1–3.

Fitzgerald F (1994) The tyranny of health. *New England Journal of Medicine.* **331**(July 21): 196–8.

Fox NJ, Ward KJ and O'Rourke AJ (2005) The 'expert patient': empowerment or medical dominance? The case of weight loss, pharmaceutical drugs and the Internet. *Social Science and Medicine.* **60**(6): 1299-309.

Frank A (1995) *The Wounded Storyteller: body, illness, and ethics.* University of Chicago Press, Chicago.

Galvin R (2002) Disturbing notions of chronic illness and individual responsibility: towards a genealogy of morals. *Health.* **6**(2): 107–37.

Garlick W (2003) *Patient Information: What's the Prognosis?* Consumer's Association, London.

Gillespie R, Florin D and Gillam S (2002) *Changing Relationship: findings from the Patient Involvement Project.* King's Fund, London, Executive summary.

Goldsmith J (1999) Patients and families as partners – sharing the burden of knowledge. *BMJ.* www.bmj.bmjjournals.com/cgi/eletters/318/7186/DC1#2547

Grime J and Pollock K (2004) Information v experience: A comparison of an information leaflet on antidepressants with lay experience of treatment. *Patient Education and Counselling.* **54**: 361–8.

Guevara JP, Wolf FM, Grum CM and Clark NM (2003) Effects of educational interventions for self management of asthma in children and adolescents: systematic review and meta-analysis. *BMJ.* **326**(14 June): 1308.

Hannay D (1979) *The Symptom Iceberg: a study of community health.* Routledge and Kegan Paul, London.

Hardey M (1999) Doctor in the house: the Internet as a source of lay health knowledge and the challenge to expertise. *Sociology of Health and Illness.* **21**(6): 820–35.

Hardey M (2002) 'The story of my illness': personal accounts of illness on the Internet. *Health.* **6**(1): 31–46.

Haynes RB (1976) Strategies for improving compliance: a methodologic analysis and review. In: DL Sackett and RB Haynes (eds) *Compliance with Therapeutic Regimes.* Johns Hopkins University Press, Baltimore, pp. 69–82.

Haynes RB (1979) Strategies to improve compliance with referrals, appointments and prescribed medical regimes. In: RB Haynes and DL Sackett (eds) *Compliance in Health Care.* Johns Hopkins University Press, Baltimore.

Haynes RB and Sackett DL (1979) *Compliance in Health Care.* Johns Hopkins University Press, Baltimore.

Heath I (2003) A wolf in sheep's clothing: a critical look at the ethics of drug taking. *BMJ*. **327**(11 October): 856–8.

Henwood F, Wyatt S, Hart A and Smith J (2003) 'Ignorance is bliss sometimes': constraints on the emergence of the 'informed patient' in the changing landscapes of health information. *Sociology of Health and Illness*. **25**(6): 589–607.

Heritage J (1997) Conversation analysis and institutional talk, analysing data. In: D Silverman (ed.) *Qualitative Research: theory, method and practice*. Sage, London, pp. 161–82.

Herxheimer A (2003) Relationships between the pharmaceutical industry and patients' organisations. *BMJ*. **326**(31 May): 1208–10.

Hope T (1996) *Evidence Based Patient Choice*. King's Fund, London.

Horne R and Weinman J (2004) The theoretical basis of concordance and issues for research. In: C Bond (ed.) *Concordance: a partnership in medicine taking*. Pharmaceutical Press, London, pp. 119–45.

Hughes CM and McCann S (2003) Perceived interprofessional barriers between community pharmacists and general practitioners: a qualitative assessment. *British Journal of General Practice*. **53**: 600–6.

Hughes L, Whittlesea C and Luscombe D (2002) Patients' knowledge and perceptions of the side-effects of OTC medication. *Journal of Clinical Pharmacy and Therapeutics*. **27**: 243–8.

Hyden, L-C (1997) Illness and narrative. *Sociology of Health and Illness*. **19**(1): 48–69.

Ingleby D (1981) *Critical Psychiatry: the politics of mental health*. Penguin, Harmondsworth.

Jacobsen B, Smith A and Whitehead M (1991) *The Nation's Health: A Strategy for the 1990s: a report from an independent multidisciplinary committee*. King Edward's Hospital Fund for London, London.

Jadad AR (1999) Promoting partnerships: challenges for the internet age. *BMJ*. **319**(18 September): 761–4.

Jaye C and Wilson H (2003) When general practitioners become patients. *Health*. **7**(2): 201–55.

Johnson JL (1991) Learning to live again: the process of adjustment following a heart attack. In: JM Morse and JL Johnson (eds) *The Illness Experience: dimensions of suffering*. Sage, London.

Johnstone L (2000) *Users and Abusers of Psychiatry*. Routledge, London.

Jones R, Finlay F, Crouch V and Anderson S (2000) Drug information leaflets: adolescent and professional perspectives. *Child: Care, Health and Development*. **26**(1): 41–8.

Jorgensen KJ and Gotzsche PC (2004) Presentation on websites of possible benefits and harms from screening for breast cancer: cross sectional study. *BMJ*. **328**(17 January): 148.

Josh VK (2003) Squamous cell carcinomas of the head and neck. *BMJ*. **326**(1 February): 282.

Kangas I (2001) Making sense of depression: perceptions of melancholia in lay narratives. *Health*. **5**(1): 76–92.

Kangas I (2002) 'Lay' and 'expert': illness knowledge constructions in the sociology of health and illness. *Health*. **6**(3): 301–4.

Keech P (2004) Telling it how it is. *BMJ*. **328**(17 April): 918.

Kendall L (2001) *The Future Patient*. IPPR, London.

Kennedy A, Robinson A and Rogers A (2003) Incorporating patients' views and experiences of life with IBS in the development of an evidence based self-help guidebook. *Patient Education and Counselling*. **50**: 303–10.

Kiley R and Graham E (2002) *The Patient's Internet Handbook*. Royal Society of Medicine Press, London.

Kilian R, Lindenbach I, Lobig U, Uhle M, Petscheleit A and Angermayer MC (2003) Indicators of empowerment and disempowerment in the subjective evaluation of the psychiatric treatment process by persons with severe and persistent mental illness: a qualitative and quantitative analysis. *Social Science and Medicine*. **56**(6): 1127–42.

Kirk P, Kirk I and Kristjanson LJ (2004) What do patients receiving palliative care for cancer and their families want to be told? A Canadian and Australian qualitative study. *BMJ*. **328**: 1343.

Kleinman A (1988) *The Illness Narratives: suffering, healing and the human condition*. Basic Books, United States.

Kmietowicz Z (2004) Admissions to hospital under the Mental Health Act rise by 30% over 10 years. *BMJ*. **328**(10): April, p. 854.

Kohner N and Hill AP (2000) *Help! Does My Patient Know More Than Me?* King's Fund, London.

Laing RD (1960) *The Divided Self*. Tavistock Publications, London.

Laing RD and Esterson A (1970) *Sanity, Madness and the Family: families of schizophrenics*. Pelican Books, London.

Lambert B (1995) Directness and deference in pharmacy students' messages to physicians. *Social Science and Medicine*. **40**(4): 545–55.

Landers M, Blenkinsopp A, Pollock K and Grime J (2002) Community pharmacists and depression: the pharmacist as intermediary between patient and doctor. *International Journal of Pharmacy Practice*. **10**: 253–65.

Launer J (2002) *Narrative-based Primary Care, a practical guide*. Radcliffe Medical Press, Oxford.

Lee-Trewick G (2001) I'm not ill, it's just this back: osteopathic treatment, responsibility and back problems. *Health*. **5**(1): 31–49.

Ley P (1982) Satisfaction, compliance and communication. *British Journal of Clinical Psychology*. **21**: 241–54.

Ley P (1997) *Communicating With Patients: improving communication, satisfaction and compliance*. Stanley Thornes (Publishers) Ltd, Cheltenham.

Ley P and Spelman MS (1967) *Communicating with the Patient*. Staples Press, London.

Leydon GM, Boulton M, Moyhihan C, Jones A, Mossman J, Boudioni M and McPherson K (2000) Cancer patients' information needs and information seeking behaviour: in depth interview study. *BMJ*. **320**(1 April): 909–13.

Lorig K (2000) Patients as partners in managing chronic disease. *BMJ*. **320**(26 February): 526–7.

Lorig K, Holman H, Sobel D, Laurent D, Gonzalez V and Minor M (1994) *Living a Healthy Life with Chronic Conditions: self-management of heart disease, arthritis, stroke, diabetes, asthma, bronchitis, emphysema and others*. Bull Publishing, Colorado.

Lupton D (1997) Consumerism, reflexivity and the medical encounter. *Social Science and Medicine*. **45**(3): 373–81.

MacPherson R, Jerrom B and Hughes A (1996) A controlled study of education about drug treatment in schizophrenia. *British Journal of Psychiatry*. **168**: 709–17.

Makoul G, Arntson P and Schofield T (1995) Health promotion in primary care: physician–patient communication and decision making about prescription medications. *Social Science and Medicine*. **41**(9): 1241–54.

Malone M, Harris R, Hooker R, Tucker T, Tanna N and Honnor S (2004) Health and the Internet – changing boundaries in primary care. *Family Practice*. **21**(2): 189–91.

McGrath JM (1999) Physicians' perspectives on communicating prescription drug information. *Qualitative Health Research*. **9**(6): 731–836.

McKinstry A and McKee M (2000) Do patients wish to be involved in decision making in the consultation? A cross sectional survey with video vignettes. *BMJ*. **321**: 867–71.

McPherson A (1999) The problem with medical advice columns. *BMJ*. **319**(2 October): 928.

Medawar C, Herxheimer A, Bell A and Jofre S (2002) Paroxetine, *Panorama* and user reporting of ADRs: Consumer intelligence matters in clinical practice and post-marketing surveillance. *International Journal of Risk and Safety in Medicine*. **15**: 161–9.

Misselbrook D (2001) *Thinking About Patients*. Petroc Press, Newbury.

Misselbrook D and Armstrong D (2001) Patients' responses to risk information about the benefits of treating hypertension. *British Journal of General Practice*. **51**: 276–9.

Moore RJ, Chamberlain RM and Khuri FR (2004) Communicating suffering in primary stage head and neck cancer. *European Journal of Cancer Care.* **13**: 53–64.

Moumjid N, Morelle M, Carrer, M-O, Bachelot T, Mignotte H and Bremond A (2003) Elaborating patient information with patients themselves: lessons from a cancer treatment focus group. *Health Expectations.* **6**: 128–39.

Nair K, Dolovich L, Cassels A, McCormack J, Levine M, Gray J, Mann K and Burns S (2002) What patients want to know about their medications. Focus group study of patient and clinician perspectives. *Canadian Family Physician.* **48**(January): 104–10.

Newnes C, Holmes G and Dunn C (1999) *This is Madness: a critical look at psychiatry and the future of mental health services.* PCCS Books, Ross-on-Wye.

Newnes C, Holmes G and Dunn C (2001) *This is Madness Too: critical perspectives on mental health services.* PCCS Books, Ross-on-Wye.

NHSCRD (2000) Informing, communicating and sharing decisions with people who have cancer. *Effective Health Care.* **6**(6): 1–8.

NICE (2002) *Schizophrenia: core interventions in the treatment and management of schizophrenia in primary and secondary care. NICE Clinical guideline.* NICE, London.

NIMHE (2003) *Self-help Interventions for Mental Health Problems.* December 2003. National Institute for Mental Health in England. www.nimhe.org.uk

Perkins R and Repper E (1999) Compliance or informed choice. *Journal of Mental Health.* **8**(2): 117–29.

Pollock K and Grime J (2004) *Meeting the Treatment Information Needs of Users of Specialist Mental Health Services. A study of users' experience of information provision within a complex system of health care.* Keele University, Department of Medicines Management.

Pollock K, Grime J, Baker E and Mantala K (2004) Meeting the information needs of psychiatric inpatients: staff and patient perspectives. *Journal of Mental Health.* **13**(4): 389–401.

Protheroe J, Fahey T, Montgomery A and Peters T (2000) The impact of patients' preferences on the treatment of atrial fibrillation: observational study of patient based decision analysis. *BMJ.* **320**: 1380–4.

Quirk A and Lelliott P (2001) What do we know about life on acute psychiatric wards in the UK? A review of the research evidence. *Social Science and Medicine.* **53**(12): 1565–74.

Radley A (1996) The critical moment: time, information and medical expertise in the experience of patients receiving coronary bypass surgery. In: S Williams and M Calnan (eds) *Modern Medicines: lay perspectives and experiences.* UCL Press, London, pp. 118–38.

Raynor DKT and Britten N (2001) Medicine information leaflets fail concordance test. *BMJ.* **322**(23 June): 1541.

Read J and Reynolds J (1996) *Speaking Our Minds: an anthology of personal experiences of mental distress and its consequences.* The Open University, Milton Keynes.

Reebye RN, Avery AJ, Bissell P and Van Weel C (2002) The issue of territoriality between pharmacists and physicians in primary care. *International Journal of Pharmacy Practice.* **10**: 69–75.

Rees CE, Ford JE and Sheard CE (2002) Evaluating the reliability of DISCERN: a tool for assessing the quality of written patient information on treatment choices. *Patient Education and Counselling.* **47**: 273–5.

Rethink, SANE, The Zito Trust and NAPICU (2004) *Behind Closed Doors: acute mental health care in the UK.* Joint Report. www.rethink.org

Richards D (2004) Self-help: empowering service users or aiding cash strapped mental health services? *Journal of Mental Health.* **13**(2): 117–23.

Richards H, Reid M and Watt G (2003) Victim-blaming revisited: a qualitative study of beliefs about illness causation, and responses to chest pain. *Family Practice.* **20**(6): 711–16.

Rogers A, Hassell K and Nikolaas G (1999) *Demanding Patients? Analysing the use of primary care.* Open University Press, Buckingham.

Rogers A, Pilgrim D and Lacey R (1993) *Experiencing Psychiatry: a users' view of services.* Macmillan/MIND, Basingstoke.

Rose D (2001) *Users' Voices: the perspectives of mental health service users on community and hospital care.* Sainsbury Centre for Mental Health, London.

Roter DL (2000) The medical visit context of treatment decision-making and the therapeutic relationship. *Health Expectations.* **3**: 17–25.

Royal College of Psychiatrists (2001) *Consultants as Partners in Care.* Royal College of Psychiatrists, London.

Rozmovits L and Ziebland S (2004) What do patients with prostate or breast cancer want from an Internet site? A qualitative study of information needs? *Patient Education and Counselling.* **53**(1): 57–64.

Rycroft-Malone J, Latter S, Yerrell P and Shaw D (2001) Consumerism in health care: the case of medication information. *Journal of Nursing Management.* **9**: 221–30.

Sackett DL (1976) Priorities and methods for future research. In: H Sackett and R Haynes (eds) *Compliance in Therapeutic Regimes.* Johns Hopkins University Press, Baltimore, pp. 169–89.

Sainsbury Centre for Mental Health (1998) *Acute Problems.* Sainsbury Centre for Mental Health, London.

Salmon P and Hall GM (2003) Patient empowerment and control: a psychological discourse in the service of medicine. *Social Science and Medicine.* **57**(10): 1969–80.

Sandvik H (1999) Health information and interaction on the internet: a survey of female urinary incontinence. *BMJ.* **319**(3 July): 29–32.

Sang B (2004) Choice, participation and accountability: assessing the potential impact of legislation promoting patient and public involvement in health in the UK. *Health Expectations.* **7**: 187–90.

Shapiro J, Mosqueda L and Botros D (2003) A caring partnership: expectations of ageing persons with disabilities for their primary care doctors. *Family Practice.* **20**(6): 635–41.

Sharkey VB (2002) Perspectives of collaboration/non-collaboration in a mental health inpatient setting. *Journal of Psychiatric and Mental Health Nursing.* **9**: 49–55.

Silverman D (1987) Coercive interpretation of the clinic: the social constitution of the Down's Syndrome child. In: D Silverman (ed.) *Communication and Medical Practice, Social Relations in the Clinic.* Sage Publications, London.

Sitzia J and Wood N (1997) Patient satisfaction: a review of issues and concepts. *Social Science and Medicine.* **45**(12): 1829–43.

Skelton A (2001) Evolution not revolution? The struggle for the recognition and development of patient education in the UK. *Patient Education and Counselling.* **44**: 23–7.

Smith G (2002a) *Mind's Policy on Primary Care.* MIND, London.

Smith P (2002b) Letters to patients: sending the right message. *BMJ.* **324**(16 March): 685.

Smith S and Henderson M (2000) What you don't know won't hurt you. Information given to patients about the side-effects of antipsychotic drugs. *Psychiatric Bulletin.* **24**: 172–4.

Stapleton H, Kirkham M and Thomas G (2002) Qualitative study of evidence based leaflets in maternity care. *BMJ.* **324**(16 March): 639.

Stevenson F, Barry C, Britten N, Barber N and Bradley C (2000) Doctor–patient communication about drugs: the evidence for shared decision making. *Social Science and Medicine.* **50**: 829–40.

Street RL (2003) Mediated consumer-provider communication in cancer care: the empowering potential of new technologies. *Patient Education and Counselling.* **50**: 99–104.

Strong P (1979) *The Ceremonial Order of the Clinic: patients, doctors and medical bureaucracies.* Routledge and Kegan Paul, London.

Sullivan M (2003) The new subjective medicine: taking the patient's point of view on health care and health. *Social Science and Medicine.* **56**(7): 1595–1604.

Szasz TS (1970) *The Manufacture of Madness.* Harper and Row, New York.

Szasz TS (1972) *The Myth of Mental Illness: foundations of a theory of personal conduct*. Paladin, London.

Tennant R (2002) *Shaping Our Lives: patient and public involvement in health: the views of health and social care users*. King's Fund, London.

Thorne S, Ternulf Nyhlin K and Paterson BL (2000) Attitudes toward patient expertise in chronic illness. *International Journal of Nursing Studies*. **37**: 303–11.

Thornton H, Edwards A and Baum M (2003) Women need better information about routine mammography. *BMJ*. **327**(12 July): 101–3.

Towle A and Godolphin W (1999) Framework for teaching and learning informed shared decision making. *BMJ*. **319**(18 September): 766–71.

Townsend P, Davidson N and Whitehead M (1990) *Inequalities in Health: the Black Report and the health divide*. Penguin, Harmondsworth.

Treacher A and Baruch G (1981) Towards a critical history of the psychiatric profession. In: D Ingleby (ed.) *Critical Psychiatry*. Penguin, Harmondsworth, pp. 120–49.

Tuckett D, Boulton M, Olson C and Williams A (1985) *Meetings Between Experts: an approach to sharing ideas in medical consultations*. Tavistock, London.

Vuckovic N and Nichter M (1997) Changing patterns of pharmaceutical practice in the United States. *Social Science and Medicine*. **44**(9): 1285–302.

Wallcroft J and Bryant M (2003) *The Mental Health Service User Movement in England*. Sainsbury Centre for Mental Health, London.

Wennberg JE, Barry MJ, Fowler FJ and Mulley A (1993) Outcomes Research, PORTs and Health Care Reform. *Annals New York Academy of Sciences*. **703**: 52–62.

West P (1976) The physician and the management of childhood epilepsy. In: M Wadsworth and D Robinson (eds) *Studies in Everyday Medical Life*. Martin Robertson, London.

Wilkinson R (1996) *Unhealthy Societies*. Routledge, London.

Williams G (1984) The genesis of chronic illness: narrative reconstruction. *Sociology of Health and Illness*. **6**: 175.

Wilson P (2002) How to find the good and avoid the bad or ugly: a short guide to tools for rating quality of health information on the internet. *BMJ*. **234**(9 March): 598–602.

Wykurz G and Kelly D (2002) Developing the role of patients as teachers: literature review. *BMJ*. **325**(12 October): 818–21.

Ziebland S, Chapple A, Dumelow C, Evans J, Prinjha S and Rozmovits L (2004) How the internet affects patients' experience of cancer: a qualitative study. *BMJ*. **328**(6 March): 564–9.

Zola IK (1975) Medicine as an institution of social control. In: C Cox and A Mead (eds) *A Sociology of Medical Practice*. Collier-Macmillan, London, pp. 170–246.

Chapter Nine

Satisfaction

A significant feature of concordance is the recognition it accords the patient perspective. Awareness of patients' understanding and experience of illness and the values and aspirations which underpin treatment preferences are seen to be central to delivery of effective healthcare. As the *process* of care, rather than its outcome, assumes increasing importance, the success of interventions comes to be determined by the subjective evaluation of patients, rather than the 'objective' measurements of clinical medicine (May *et al.* 2004; Sullivan 2003). Patient satisfaction has developed as a legitimate outcome as well as a proxy indicator of the quality of care (Kelstrup *et al.* 1993; Stallard 1996; Williams 1994; Williams & Wilkinson 1995). A concern with the reflexive modification of services in response to consumer feedback developed from the managerial reforms of the Griffiths report of 1983 (Callan & Littlewood 1988; DHSS 1983; McIver 1991; Sitzia & Wood 1997). Patient-centred medicine has become the central policy commitment in a system supposedly focused on individual choice and reflexive sensitivity to patient preferences and satisfaction with care (Department of Health 1999, 2000, 2001, 2003). It is also widely assumed that satisfied 'customers' will be more highly motivated and compliant with treatment regimes, leading in turn to improved outcomes and a more cost-effective use of resources (Callan & Littlewood 1988; Crawford & Kessel 1999; Williams 1994).

Patient satisfaction surveys have been frequently employed as a quick and convenient method of obtaining an 'objective' measurement of patients' views – usually quite positive – about many aspects of healthcare. However, there is widespread agreement that such simple self-completion questionnaires over-estimate the extent of patient satisfaction with services, and that they constitute an inappropriate method for assessing a complex concept relating to a very diverse range of experiences (Avis, Bond & Arthur 1997; Calnan 1998; Crawford & Kessel 1999; McIver 1991; Sitzia & Wood 1997; Stallard 1996; Williams 1994). Such studies reflect professional judgements about how patient satisfaction is configured, and are often more or less explicitly linked to an interest in increasing compliance (Ley 1982). The selection and framing of questions directs and constrains the content of respondents' answers, effectively censoring the responses they can make (Calnan 1998; Crawford & Kessel 1999; Stallard 1996).

Satisfaction surveys have been popular because they appear to focus on patient concerns, and to be providing an opportunity to involve patients in service assessment and development, whilst actually evading engagement with the complex and ambiguous nature of patients' experience and assessment of care. Since the term lacks adequate or consistent definition, it is not clear what the results of satisfaction surveys are indicating. Where patients are encouraged to express their views in qualitative studies, their responses are consistently more negative and complex (Avis, Bond & Arthur 1997; Calnan 1998; Crawford & Kessel 1999; Edwards, Staniszweska & Crichton 2004; Letendre 1997; Mulcahy & Tritter 1998; Rogers, Pilgrim & Lacey 1993; Stallard 1996; Williams 1994; Williams & Wilkinson 1995). The significance of methodology in shaping results was clearly established in a study by Williams *et al.*, in which both quantitative and qualitative methods were used to investigate the experience of satisfaction with the same respondents (Williams, Coyle & Healy 1998).

There are many reasons why patients' expressed satisfaction is not a good indicator of the quality of service, or a valid representation of their experience and assessment of care. Patients may articulate the views they feel to be appropriate, out of gratitude or loyalty to particular professionals, or because they find it difficult to be critical of personnel and services on whom they depend for care (Calnan 1998; Rees Lewis 1994). Declared satisfaction may be an expression of support or confidence in the system, rather than the outcome of a considered process of evaluation (Williams 1994; Williams & Wilkinson 1995). It may also result from a widely reported fear of professional retribution, and patients' desire to avoid the negative attributions and stigma which complaints often attract (Coyle 1999; Sinding 2003). 'Satisfaction' is not a unitary, exclusive or stable concept (Rees Lewis 1994; Stallard 1996). People may be satisfied with some aspects of care, but not with others. Their assessments may change over time, as they reappraise the situation in the light of further information and experience (Avis, Bond & Arthur 1997; Stimson & Webb 1975). As a result, negative feelings and emotions may be consolidated into overt dissatisfaction and complaint, or dissipated as they are reformulated in terms of wider considerations and mitigating circumstances (Coyle 1999). Evaluation of care is likely to be influenced by outcome: if people get better they are more likely to feel satisfied with the service. Satisfaction may be an expression of health outcome rather than healthcare (Jackson, Chamberlin & Kroenke 2001).

Satisfaction has also been linked to expectations, and the relative discrepancy between patients' aspirations and their experience of care (Williams *et al.* 1995). In this case, positive satisfaction could be expressed alongside low expectations and poor services. At the outset, people may not have any particular expectations of care. These may be formulated in the light of reflection and experience (Stallard 1996; Williams & Wilkinson 1995). Avis *et al.* found that patients tended to be tentative in their expectations of what their first outpatient appointment would involve. The majority (85%) expressed satisfaction with the consultation, even though a substantial minority (38%) also acknowledged that they had been disappointed by some aspect of this. Characteristic responses at this point were relief that the consultation was over, and that their problem was now being actively investigated and addressed. However, patients brought a more evaluative and critical perspective to bear at the time of the follow-up interview. Satisfaction at this point was bound up with their assessments of the effectiveness of care, and whether or not they felt they had been adequately informed, and understood enough about their illness and treatment. A third of patients who experienced the outcome of their service contact as inconclusive felt they had been excluded from the discussion of their illness and treatment. Denied the information necessary to understand their situation, these patients were becoming resentful and critical of perceived shortcomings in the care they had received (Avis, Bond & Arthur 1997).

A number of studies have considered the processes and circumstances by which negative experiences of healthcare tend to be dissipated and deflected, rather than formulated as criticism or complaint (Mulcahy & Tritter 1998; Sinding 2003). Williams *et al.* have suggested that patient satisfaction is bound up with the evaluation of duty and culpability in relation to service provision. Where patients perceive that the system has failed in its duty of care they are likely to regard lapses as culpable. However, where untoward events can be explained in terms of mitigating circumstances services and staff will not be held responsible (Edwards, Staniszweska & Crichton 2004; Williams, Coyle & Healy 1998). Edwards *et al.* identified several reasons why respondents in their sample of patients undergoing orthopaedic surgery did not formulate disappointing or negative experiences as dissatisfaction and complaint. Patients were reluctant to criticise staff on whom they depended for ongoing care. In addition, dwelling on the past, and perpetuating the negative experiences associated with it, was not compatible with the positive outlook which they preferred to maintain. The personal cost of pursuing dissatisfaction may be considerable – in terms of time, effort and frustration – for no very clear or tangible gain. Respondents often had no wish to dwell on, and so amplify, the impact of earlier disappointments which were felt to hinder the process of recovery and readjustment following surgery (Edwards, Staniszweska & Crichton 2004).

The personal cost of harbouring dissatisfaction, and consequent disinclination to do so, is strikingly illustrated in Sinding's study of 12 carers of patients who had died of breast cancer (Sinding 2003). Negative experiences of distress, suffering and inadequate care were described by all the carers. However, respondents took account of mitigating circumstances in excusing staff from responsibility for shortcomings in the provision of care. Cancer was perceived to be a particularly deadly illness, beyond the bounds of professional expertise to control and treat effectively. Additionally, where staff were perceived to be working in difficult circumstances and doing their best with inadequate resources they were exonerated from blame. Paradoxically, Sinding found that respondents' accounts of intensely distressing experiences could also be associated with positive responses and evaluation. One of her respondents described the gruelling experience his wife had undergone shortly before her death when she had been kept for 30 hours on an emergency ward trolley just a few days after undergoing surgery on her back. Afterwards, he wrote a letter to the ward staff thanking them, and trying to express his appreciation for their care, 'Because they did everything they possibly could' (Sinding 2003 p. 1381). In a situation which others might well have defined as grossly negligent the respondent accepts that the hospital was simply unable to provide a bed for his desperately sick wife and, consequently, there were no grounds for complaint. Sinding observes that, especially in cases where death rendered complaints beyond redress, relatives may have good reason not to formulate or pursue grievances. In a fundamental sense, this was recognised to be pointless, and also personally damaging. Dwelling on unpleasant events could intensify the distress of bereavement, preventing closure or the positive reconstruction of final memories of the deceased. The possibility of different outcomes, that death might have been avoided had care been managed differently, was a deeply distressing prospect, and a spur to such 'functional avoidance' (Mulcahy & Tritter 1998), particularly as it would implicate the surviving carer in the inadequacy of care. 'Disarming' complaints in this way may be adaptive for the individual, but dysfunctional for the system as a whole, allowing unsatisfactory care to pass unchallenged and uncorrected (Sinding 2003).

Stimson and Webb observed that patients were reluctant to voice direct complaints about their medical care. However, they contrasted the passive demeanour usually exhibited in the consulting room with the much livelier, and critical, accounts patients often constructed afterwards. Such 'atrocity stories' are a response to conflict or dissatisfaction with medical encounters. They constitute a partial redress for the subordinate role the patient is constrained to adopt during the consultation, and a reassertion of his personal integrity and competency afterwards. Such stories provide a medium through which complaints may be formulated and grievances aired informally and in the process, also, defused (Stimson & Webb 1975). It is apparent that in relation to the frequency of patients' experienced disappointment with healthcare, formal complaints are rare and unusual events (Mulcahy & Tritter 1998). Sinding's study shows that people are prepared to tolerate even gross lapses in standards of service, provided they retain confidence in the competence and motivation of the staff involved in providing care (Sinding 2003). However, Coyle's analysis indicates that what often tips the balance for patients in turning negative experiences of healthcare into overt dissatisfaction is the affront that results from dealing with insensitive services and discourteous staff and the loss of self-esteem and sense of disempowerment that results from this (Coyle 1999). Such 'personal identity threats' are deeply offensive. It may be that when people say they are dissatisfied with health services they are primarily expressing their dissatisfaction with their relationships and the quality of communication with the professionals they have encountered throughout their experience of care.

'Satisfaction' remains an elusive concept, complex and hard to capture or evaluate. It is not necessarily a marker of quality care or of services which adequately provide for patients' preferences and needs. As with other currently fashionable terms denoting 'patient-centredness', such as 'patient choice', 'information needs' and 'shared decision making', 'patient satisfaction' is a professional construct, without particular relevance or resonance for patients. Over and over again, however, research has revealed that when they are ill, and in addition to receiving effective medical treatment, what people want most of all is simply to be treated with understanding and compassion. Patients strive, often unsuccessfully, to be treated as an individual, rather than a 'case' (Coyle 1999; Shapiro, Mosqueda & Botros 2003; Sitzia & Wood 1997) and to feel that professionals have properly understood their concerns and *acknowledged* their suffering (Beach *et al.* 2005; Bissell, May & Noyce 2004; Calnan & Williams 1996; Cape 2001; Gask *et al.* 2003; Kleinman 1988; Stimson & Webb 1975; Williams *et al.* 1995).

Patients endeavour to retain professional approval out of a desire to avoid alienation, but also because they value the intrinsically therapeutic effects of good relationships. To a great extent, patients are committed to being satisfied with the care they receive, because they *need* to trust the competence of the professionals on whom they depend for help (Salkeld *et al.* 2004). Reassurance is an important goal, and often a sufficient reason for patients to consult (Britten 1994; Britten 2004; Donovan & Blake 2000; Edwards *et al.* 2001). A study of patients referred for specialist investigation of arthritis revealed that the achievement of effective reassurance depended on respondents' perception that their doctors had heard and properly acknowledged their difficulties and concerns (Donovan & Blake 2000). Salkeld *et al.* reported that regardless of their stated preferences for involvement in decision making, trust in their surgeon was a priority for patients undergoing surgery for colorectal cancer and essential to accepting that the right treatment decision had been made. Trust was generated by confidence in professional expertise and also by the surgeon's capacity to convey an impression of genuine concern about the patient. This was expressed by taking time to provide information and also to acknowledge and discuss patients' anxieties and questions in a respectful and empathetic manner. Even patients who expressed a desire for involvement in decision making relied on their doctor's opinion, and sought to understand the basis for professional judgement rather than to take direct responsibility for treatment decisions themselves (Salkeld *et al.* 2004).

Eliciting patients' perspectives demonstrates professional respect and interest, opens up scope for patient participation and contributes to the realisation of a 'therapeutic alliance', a major goal of concordant consultations (Frankel & Beckman 1989). Alongside the recurring finding that patients consistently value good relationships with professionals based on the qualities of respect, empathy and consideration, there is considerable evidence that their aspirations are frequently disappointed (Beach *et al.* 2005; Cox *et al.* 2004; Meredith 1993; Shapiro, Mosqueda & Botros 2003; Tate 2003). Meredith found that neither patients nor surgeons experienced outpatient clinic consultations as an appropriate vehicle for effective communication and that they were operating with very different perceptions of its proper purpose and function. Surgeons regarded the consultation to be concerned primarily with technical and instrumental aspects of diagnosis and treatment. Patients viewed it as an opportunity for explanation and communication, and felt disvalued and discouraged by the cursory and impersonal way in which they felt they were treated (Meredith 1993). Other studies and reviews have commented on the lack of empathy, interest and understanding that doctors routinely express towards patients in medical consultations (Cox *et al.* 2004; Tate 2003). In a detailed analysis of verbal and non-verbal communication between patients and doctors in a cancer clinic, Beach *et al.* have shown how professionals routinely evade patients' expressions of fear and uncertainty. Cues and invitations to address psychosocial issues and concerns are rejected through the unresponsive and non-empathetic pursuit of a narrow technical and biomedical agenda. In this way, the opportunity to establish an effective therapeutic alliance is repeatedly squandered (Beach *et al.* 2005).

It has been argued that time constraints are a major factor limiting the realisation of patient-centred consultations (Howie *et al.* 1999; Martin *et al.* 1999; Roland *et al.* 1986). Against this, it has been suggested that good communication does not necessarily take longer, and may even save time, in contributing to more effective use of resources, and reducing the number of follow-up consultations (Knight 1987; Ogden *et al.* 2004; Pollock & Grime 2002; Tuckett *et al.* 1985; Williams & Neal 1998). There is no clear relationship between the length and quality of medical consultations (Carr-Hill *et al.* 1998; Clark & Gong 2000; Epstein 2000; Morrell *et al.* 1986; Tate 2003; Towle & Godolphin 1999; Tuckett *et al.* 1985; Wiggers & Sanson-Fisher 1997; Wilson 1991). What seems to be important is not the actual length of the consultation, but the capacity of professionals to convey the *impression* that the patient has enough time to tell his story, express his concerns and discuss the relevant options for treatment. Edwards *et al.* found that within the acknowledged constraints of time shortage and limited personal knowledge, patients did not necessarily regard it as appropriate or possible that they should take an active role in making clinical decisions about care and treatment. However, they wanted to feel that they were able to make a contribution to the consultation, had been presented with all relevant options, and had been treated respectfully and as an equal. Thus, it is the *feeling* of being informed and involved in decision making, and the *sense* of not being hurried that are critical in determining patients' sense of being appropriately involved in the consultation (Edwards *et al.* 2001). In a similar way, Burkitt-Wright *et al.* describe how the *manner* in which doctors explained their illness and treatment options was of greater significance for breast cancer patients than the amount of information they received, or the extent to which they exercised genuine choice of treatment. In particular, the feeling that they had been presented with an *option* was important, even if, in practice, all respondents acceded to their doctors' recommendations. In this context, framing the preferred clinical choice as an option which women had a theoretical and acknowledged entitlement to reject served as a marker or respect and acknowledgement of the patient's autonomy, rather than constituting an opportunity for active choice and the assumption of responsibility for treatment (Burkitt Wright, Holcombe & Salmon 2004).

These studies illustrate that it is not so much the information that is conveyed but the understanding that is negotiated that is important in determining the success of the consultation. The promise of concordance lay in its potential to open up professional awareness of the nature of patient perspectives and the importance of addressing these directly through its incorporation within the mainstream policy agenda. However, the ideas and insights of 'concordance' are far from new. The significance of patients' experience and understanding of illness has been articulated in an extensive body of writing and research from the 1960s onwards (Balint 1957). The shift in focus from the biomedical agenda to the exploration of patient subjectivity is expressed in the now well established distinction between 'disease' and 'illness' (Eisenberg 1978). 'Disease' refers to the observable manifestions of organic pathology, the conventional objects of clinical scrutiny and evaluation. 'Illness' refers to the subjective experience of malfunction and malaise, which is shaped by personal and cultural interpretation and attribution. Disease and illness do not necessarily coincide e.g. as in the case of asymptomatic conditions such as hypertension, or 'functional' disorders such as chronic pain, ME or fibromyalgia. Most psychiatric diagnoses similarly lack any biological underpinning (Boyle 1990; Bracken & Thomas 2001; Eisenberg 1978; Kutchins & Kirk 1999; Szasz 1970).

Kleinman has proposed that for medical interventions to be successful, clinicians must deal effectively with illness as well as disease. In pursuing a single-minded focus on the recognition and treatment of disease, however, biomedicine has largely written out the nature and significance of illness, and the patient's experience of suffering. Consequently, it has been unable to deal adequately with many of the most prevalent causes of morbidity affecting the populations of modern industrial societies. These are characterised by a high incidence of psychosocial distress, either freestanding or occurring as a component of the experience of chronic illness and enduring disability.

In the narrow biological terms of the biomedical model, . . . disease is reconfigured only as an alteration in biological structure or functioning. When chest pain can be reduced to a treatable acute lobar pneumonia, this biological reductionism is an enormous success. When chest pain is reduced to chronic coronary artery disease for which calcium blockers and nitroglycerine are prescribed, while the patient's fear, the family's frustration, the job conflict, the sexual impotence, and the financial crisis go undiagnosed and unaddressed, it is a failure.

Kleinman (1988: 5–6)

In many cases, where recovery is not a realistic option, the most significant and effective contribution that health professionals can make is to assist patients in dealing with the emotional distress and anxiety that inevitably accompany intractable problems and enduring disability. Such interventions relate predominantly to the recognition and understanding of patients' experience of illness, rather than the biomedical treatment of disease. Disparity, and even conflict, between lay and professional understandings and interpretation of illness are themselves a frequent cause of patient distress and dissatisfaction with clinical encounters. Effective clinical communication can reduce the distance between the explanatory models which patients and doctors construct about illness. However, this is only possible if professionals are made aware of the significance of patients' experience of illness, and are willing and able to explore the personal and cultural meanings that attach to this (Kleinman 1980, 1988).

The recognition of patient subjectivity and the need to devise more effective methods of providing support to those suffering from chronic conditions and enduring disability has generated an interest in patient narratives (Bury 2001; Elwyn & Gwyn 1999; Frank 1995; Good 1994; Heath 1998; Hyden 1997; Kangas 2001; Launer 2003; Radley 1993; Williams 1984). The stories people tell provide a powerful mechanism for illuminating the experience of illness. Bury characterised the effect of serious illness as a 'biographical disruption', threatening social and personal identity, as well as the physical integrity, of the person (Bury 1982). Williams described the process of 'narrative reconstruction' through which people attempt to make sense of illness by reframing experience to link the wider scheme or project of their lives (Williams 1984). Similarly, Blaxter and Paterson noted that respondents in their study of working class women attempted to link together the occurrence of significant life events and the subsequent experience of illness in their lives, as a means of presenting an integrated and meaningful account which reduced the recognition and significance of contingency (Blaxter & Paterson 1982; Blaxter 1983, 1993).

Illness explanations confer meaning on otherwise arbitrary and inchoate experiences. Fashioning coherence in this way can enable a sense of control to be established, albeit precariously. Narrative seeks to repair the disruption of life occasioned by illness, and to account for 'the particularity of misfortune' (Evans-Pritchard 1937). Medical narratives, in contrast, often have no 'meaning' for the patient's experience of illness: they cannot account for *why* illness strikes: for the patient, *how* is usually a much lesser consideration. Illness narratives articulate personal explanatory models which draw on, and contribute to, cultural forms for the communication and expression of distress, and the appropriate manner of response to suffering (Hyden 1997; Kleinman 1980, 1988; Morris 1998). Narratives are tailored for particular purposes and revised in the light of experience and reflection. Frank discusses three generic types of narrative, any or all of which may be used by the same individual in different contexts and stages of illness (Frank 1995). The restitution narrative tells how the experience of illness was resolved by successful treatment and recovery: the individual is restored to health. The chaos narrative is, in contrast, an anti-narrative, lacking a structure, progression or sequence: it articulates the disintegration of the self precipitated by the experience of the body out of control. The quest narrative proposes that the challenge of illness may be self-enhancing, through the insight and character forged by suffering.

Restitution narratives are the dominant and culturally preferred form of illness story in modernist society. In addition to the intrinsic desire for health restored, they express an ideological commitment to containing illness through the technical mastery and scientific control of the material world. The medical narrative of restitution depicts the professional as actively heroic, while the passive patient fulfils his responsibility through stoic obedience and compliance. Frank comments that Parsons' model of the sick role represents a sociological form of the restitution narrative. Its resonance as a master narrative for how the relations between the sick and the well, patients and professionals, *should* be conducted accounts for its continuing influence, despite the considerable distance between model and reality. In contrast to restitution stories, quest narratives downplay the role of medicine. The patient occupies centre stage in the effort to transcend the experience of illness and in the process to resist the 'colonisation' of institutional medicine. Restitution narratives aim to reassure, and quest narratives to inspire. However, chaos narratives are universally disturbing in their revelation of human vulnerability and exposure of professional failure.

It is in the telling of stories about illness that memory is *created*, rather than recorded (Frank 1995). In addition to explaining illness, stories also provide a means of communicating and sharing experience: they are the product of the interaction between the speaker and his audience (family, friends, fellow patient, professional). Narrative has been proposed as an important tool of patient-centred medicine, with obvious relevance to concordance. Being listened to, and feeling understood, is powerful therapy. Kleinman proposes that often the greatest professional contribution to patient wellbeing may be the 'empathic witnessing', and consequent legitimation, of patients' accounts of illness and associated suffering (Kleinman 1980, 1988). Frank emphasises the significance of illness narratives as *testimony* and their *witnessing* as an ethical imperative. This obligation on the part of the well is balanced by the pedagogical functions of illness narratives in expanding lay and professional insight into the experience of sickness and the complexity of treatment decisions. These need always to be anchored in the particularity of individual circumstances and aspirations. Accepting the pedagogical contribution of testimony is important also in restoring agency to the ill, because:

> People whose reality is denied can remain recipients of treatments and services, but they cannot be participants in empathic relations of care.
>
> Frank (1995: 109)*

* Frank A (1995) Reproduced with permission from The University of Chicago Press, Chicago, IL.

Morris makes the point more forcefully:

> There are few clearer ways to express disrespect for other people than not to listen to what they say.
>
> Morris (1998: 263)*

Nevertheless, as was evident from the discussion in Chapter 6, the perpetuation of deeply entrenched traditional roles of patient and professional and the bureaucratic format effectively suppress patients' capacity to tell their stories or express their concerns in conventional consultations (Beach *et al.* 2005; Beckman & Frankel 1984; Kettunen *et al.* 2001; Kleinman 1988; Marvel *et al.* 1999; Misselbrook 2001; Strong 1979). Structured asymmetry and professional dominance legitimate the breaking of conventional norms of conversational politeness. Patients' accounts are truncated, interrupted and corrupted as material for a stereotypical 'case' or medical record over which they have no control or input. Illness narratives are routinely ignored by professionals in search of 'evidence' and the pursuit of 'best' clinical practice. In addition, it is difficult for patients to resist the professional narratives imposed upon them, especially when these involve the application of labels (such as 'depression', 'ME' or 'fibromyalgia'), which in sticking fast pathologise experience and undermine esteem, both social and personal. Far from being alleviated, the distress occasioned by 'living a life of overwhelming trouble and suffering' (Frank 1995: 112) is amplified and prolonged.

Illness experiences which cannot be accommodated within restitution narratives which affirm the power and success of medical practice and professional expertise are subject to censure and stigma. People whose problems are not resolved, who consult frequently and 'inappropriately', are likely to attract negative stereotypes as difficult, demanding, malingering, neurotic or even 'hateful' patients (Butler & Evans 1999; Dixon-Woods & Critchley 1999; Gerrard & Riddell 1988; Groves 1978; O'Dowd 1988; Raine *et al.* 2004; Roth 1986; Werner & Malterud 2003; White 2002). Those who fail to conform to the role of the (reasonably) 'good' patient are likely to be construed as inadequate, non-compliant and the author of their own misfortunes (Bissell 2003; Fitzgerald 1994; Galvin 2002; Giacomini *et al.* 2001). There is evidence that patients themselves are coming to internalise such attributions of responsibility and blame for illness and that this impacts negatively on their willingness to seek professional care (Richards, Reid & Watt 2003).

Linking health and lifestyle presents illness as substantially a matter of *choice*. This is very clearly expressed in recent policy documents and statements which emphasise the extent of personal responsibility for illness and effectively equate health with competence (Department of Health 2003, 2005).

> Self-efficacy also predicts a healthy lifestyle. The philosophy which underlies the expert patient programme has implications for the ways in which people live their lives beyond just the management of chronic disease. Those who are able to deal successfully with the problems posed by a chronic illness, and those who avoid illness through a positive lifestyle, may have a great deal in common. Such people live longer and healthier and are an example of how more

* From DB Morris *Illness and Culture in the Postmodern Age.* © 1998 The Regents of the University of California.

assertive engagement with one's own health and with the healthcare system can improve both the length and the quality of people's lives.

Donaldson (2003: 1279)*

The goal of healthcare becomes that of 'empowering' people to take responsibility for illness. 'Information' is regarded as a core component in developing patient expertise, and shifting the burden of healthcare from state to consumer. The expert patient is trained in accordance with the best evidence available to clinical medicine, from which it is assumed that a commitment to professional rationality will follow. Exercising choice to realise health equates to acting in accordance with official prescriptions. 'Empowerment' effectively equates with submission to the discipline of (informed) compliance. This marks the continuation of a persistent tendency in both professional medicine and government health policy to ignore the great extent to which health is situationally embedded in the wider contexts of people's lives, and the economic and social factors which constrain their chances and choices relating to life and health (Bissell, May & Noyce 2004; Blaxter 1982; Cornwell 1985; Galvin 2002; Richards, Reid & Watt 2003). Individualising illness, and identifying the individual as the locus of control and responsibility for misfortune, conveniently deflects attention from the wider issues of social and economic inequality and their importance in generating and maintaining inequalities in health (Jacobsen, Smith & Whitehead 1991; Townsend, Davidson & Whitehead 1990; Townsend, Phillimore & Beattie 1988; Wilkinson 1996).

In practice, 'patient choice' and the commitment to 'patient-centred medicine' have become circumscribed by dominant professional and policy paradigms linking responsibility and entitlement. There is no room here for patient expertise as a means of *resistance* to professional dominance or the basis of alternative choices as an expression of different treatment goals and preferred health outcomes. Nor is there receptiveness to the value of patient narratives as a pedagogical resource and source of insight for professionals. Instead, the preoccupation with 'educating' patients to perform more effectively within the terms of the clinical paradigm and professional rationality continues to be expressed through an industry of production and distribution of patient information materials. Concordance, which once promised so much more, has substantially been co-opted as a pseudonym for 'compliance' (Armstrong 2005; Heath 2003; Shaw 2004). The Medicines Partnership Task Force was set up by the Department of Health in 2002 to develop the practical implementation and dissemination of the concept of concordance (www.medicines-partnership.org). In the main, however, its activities express a narrow focus on the goal of educating (equated to 'empowering') patients about medicines, as a means of encouraging their more compliant, or at least less wasteful, and more cost-effective consumption: this is the bottom line on which concordance has to deliver (Shaw 2004). In this perspective, concordance is not mistaken for compliance, but it is seen to be an instrument of its realisation. Information is valued as a tool for enabling patients to understand the purpose of medicines and how to use them and to be able to discuss such matters intelligently in medical consultations. This enables professionals to become aware of patient concerns and misconceptions and,

* Donaldson L (2003) Reproduced with permission from the BMJ Publishing Group.

consequently, to dispel them (Horne & Weinman 2004). Once this is achieved, compliance is assumed, at least on the part of the rational and responsible. Education is an entitlement supporting patient 'empowerment', enabling the active 'choice' of health, and justifying the current bombardment of patients with education. Information, in effect, is valued as a means of 'training' consumers to become better patients, within the biomedical paradigm. However, as health is increasingly linked to lifestyle, entitlement to medical care is coming to be justified in relation to personal responsibility (Department of Health 2003, 2005). Information is thus being harnessed as a disciplinary medium in the reconfiguration of the patient role from passive recipient of care, to active entrepreneur of health. Illness is coming increasingly to be assessed as a mark of incompetence rather than misfortune (Fitzgerald 1994; Galvin 2002). All this is being accomplished within a formal rhetoric of patient 'choice' and 'empowerment' and increased professional responsiveness and accountability.

The modern myths of 'patient choice' and 'empowerment' reinforce the traditional goals of biomedicine as a form of restitution narrative. The discipline of healthy lifestyle and compliance with expert professional advice ensure the maintenance or restoration of health, which are construed as the outcome of personal choice and control. The common reality of illness as arbitrary, inexorable, overwhelming and terminal does not feature in this schema. The image of the informed and active patient does not give space to the recognition of pain, anxiety, vulnerability, dependency and confusion as intrinsic to the experience of illness. The highly educated citizens of modern industrial societies, in which a preoccupation with health has become something of a fetish, are often willing to embrace health maintenance as an active project, and to desire a relatively high level of information about specific illnesses that confront them. Nevertheless, the preceding discussion has reviewed a considerable amount of evidence that far from being concerned with exercising their rights of active citizenship, when people fall ill they want most of all to be treated with sympathy and consideration. The relationships they establish (or not) with those who provide professional care, and the understanding which can be brought to bear on the experience of illness as an event of personal significance, are often more important than the acquisition of technical knowledge and expertise. Rather than relishing the opportunity to demonstrate their autonomy, patients appreciate being acknowledged with professional respect and courtesy. Instead of being handed an instruction manual, they prefer to meet with support and practical help. Those who have to contend with the continuing challenges and difficulties of chronic illness or disability seek to contain these in such a way that they minimise their disruption to wider goals and commitments to which they accord a higher priority.

An irony of the drive to achieve 'patient-centred medicine' and the realisation of 'patient choice' is that, far from a responsive tailoring of care to individual circumstances, (expert) patients are being channelled into a role of standardisation and constraint. In its original conception, concordance involved the *exchange* of views between patients and professionals and, consequently, an expanded understanding of both. The consultation was recognised as a transaction, and the focus on the patient contribution served to reduce the structured asymmetry of the traditional paternalistic encounter. This view of concordance was centred on the quality of the relationship between patient and professional. The goal was to foster a therapeutic alliance based on mutual understanding and a process of negotiation which recognised the salience and individuality of patient perspectives and preferences for treatment. Kleinman has given an exemplary account of such a process (by another name) in his depiction of the 'explanatory model technique' (Kleinman 1988). Firstly, the professional elicits the patient's explanatory model of illness. In subsequently presenting his own, he engages in 'an act of translation' which if successful puts the patient in a position to actively contribute to the therapeutic process. The third stage of the process involves negotiation: 'nothing more effectively empowers patients' (Kleinman 1988: 242). This involves the doctor being frank about his own uncertainty, and also demonstrating his respect for the patient's point of view. Though not inevitable, negotiation is likely to result in compromise, and a positive and acceptable outcome to the consultation.

In Kleinman's formulation the patient is recognised as possessing an *alternate* form of knowledge, rather than inadequate scientific information. The explanatory model technique involves an act of translation, not substitution, as in the 'medicines partnership' model. The patient and professional collaborate in the formulation of an improved story of the illness and how it might be coped with (Eisenberg 1981; Heath 1998; Hyden 1997; Launer 2002). Patients are enabled to exert some choice over the type of story they construct, and the way their illness is defined (e.g. as a clinical or psychosocial problem) and to keep open options for subsequent revision. Kleinman's model focuses on the importance of shared understandings between patient and professional and the translation of meaning as a determinant of success in therapeutic encounters. It creates a space for patient and clinical expertise to coexist and for the purpose and adequacy of biomedical narratives to scrutinised. In contrast, in restricting concordance specifically to the prescribing and taking of medicines, the medicines partnership model (reflecting the policy concerns from which it derives its brief (Shaw 2004)) aligns itself squarely with the goals of biomedicine and the privileging of professional know-ledge and expertise. Effectively, concordance is reduced to a process of educating patients to achieve increased compliance and, through this, deliver a more cost-effective use of medicines. This simplified schema ignores the extent to which medicines are frequently harmful or ineffective, and closes down the opportunity that concordance originally presented for a wider consideration of medicines use and the extent to which these have become personally as well as socially problem-atic (*see* Chapter 4) (Asscher, Parr & Whitmarsh 1995; Chetley 1990; Cohen *et al.* 2001; Dieppe *et al.* 2004; Edwards 1999; Gabe & Bury 1996; Harrison & New 2002; Heath 2003; Institute of Medicine 2000; Kawachi & Conrad 1996; Medawar 1997; Petit-Zeman, Sandamas & Hogman 2001; Pirmohamed *et al.* 2004; Stricker & Psaty 2004; Vandenbrouke 2004; Vuckovic & Nichter 1997).

Given the original emphasis on concordance as an outcome of the *relationship* between doctor and patient, its subsequent restriction to the narrower instrumental focus on the prescribing and taking of medicines is unsatisfactory and disappointing. To the extent that the success of a consultation depends on the achievement of a sufficiently shared understanding between doctor and patient, then decisions about medicines as one treatment option (albeit the most frequently considered) are subsumed within the wider context of the encounter as a whole. Thus 'concordant' decisions about medicines depend on, and arise from, the success of the communication which has gone before. It does not make sense to segregate one component of a consultation as 'concordant', or ignore the extent to which successful (concordant) consultations may take place in which medicines do not feature as a topic for discussion. More significantly, in buying in to the triumphalist vision of biomedicine as routinely successful in treating disease (if only patients took their medicines as prescribed), and professional expertise as unerringly competent, the patient contribution to medical consultations continues to be obscured.

The picture of the modern patient as actively seeking information, empowerment and to be involved in medical decision making has not found extensive empirical support. In contrast, and as evidenced in the preceding discussion, patients generally continue to reproduce a role of passive deference in medical consultations. It remains difficult for both patients and professionals to transcend the organisational and interactive constraints of the bureaucratic format of the medical consultation (*see* Chapter 6). Rather than having any particular salience for the majority of patients, terms such as 'empowerment', 'shared decision making', 'patient satisfaction', 'patient-centred medicine' and even 'concordance' are professional constructs. The constitution of the patient as a reflexive consumer (Lupton 1997) expresses a mixture of academic, professional and policy interests and preoccupations – some of which are undoubtedly well intentioned and well meaning – but they do not (yet) seem to have much resonance for patients. A pragmatic concern with the cost-effective use of medicines, and the rational deployment of scarce resources is entirely appropriate and reasonable. However, it does not sit easily alongside a stated commitment to concordance as a novel paradigm of patient-centred care, requiring a wholesale change in professional culture and a different way of relating to patients. A genuinely patient-centred practice would start from a consideration of what patients themselves say they value most from medical treatment and consultations. Aside from the obvious desire to receive effective treatment, and achieve recovery, it appears that most patients prioritise establishing good relationships with health professionals, in which they feel they are treated with empathy, kindness and respect. They value the awareness of being understood, and that their concerns and suffering have been acknowledged. Thus, it is the sense of being recognised and treated as an individual, rather than a standardised, anonymous case, that seems to be one of the most important determinants of patients' assessment of the quality of care. This is not to say that people do not value information, or the opportunity to play an active part in the self-management of illness. However, particularly when they are preoccupied with the experience of pain, distress, uncertainty and fear, it is apparent that most patients do not rush to occupy the role of reflexive consumer. To the extent that the concept of concordance has been formatted in terms of the medicines partnership model involving a technical problem of patient information deficit, rather than the shared understanding of *illness*, it represents a lost opportunity to extend professional and political awareness of the dynamics of effective, humane and genuinely patient-centred, medical practice.

References

Armstrong D (2005) The myth of concordance: response to Stevenson and Scambler. *Health*. **9**(1): 23–7.

Asscher AW, Parr GD and Whitmarsh VB (1995) Towards the safer use of medicines. *BMJ.* **311**(14 October): 1003–5.

Avis M, Bond M and Arthur A (1997) Questioning patient satisfaction: an empirical investigation in two outpatient clinics. *Social Science and Medicine.* **44**(1): 85–92.

Balint M (1957) *The Doctor, His Patient, and the Illness.* Pitman Medical, London.

Beach WA, Easter DW, Good JS and Pigeron E (2005) Disclosing and responding to cancer 'fears' during oncology interviews. *Social Science and Medicine.* **60**: 893–910.

Beckman HB and Frankel RM (1984) The effect of physician behavior on the collection of data. *Annals of Internal Medicine.* **101**: 692–6.

Bissell P (2003) Compliance, concordance and respect for the patient's agenda. *Pharmaceutical Journal.* **271**(11 October): 498–500.

Bissell P, May C and Noyce PR (2004) From compliance to concordance: barriers to accomplishing a re-framed model of health care interactions. *Social Science and Medicine.* **58**: 851–62.

Blaxter M (1982) *Mothers and Daughters: a three generation study of health attitudes and behaviour.* Heinemann Educational Books, London.

Blaxter M (1983) The causes of disease: women talking. *Social Science and Medicine.* **17**(2): 59–69.

Blaxter M (1993) Why do the victims blame themselves? In: A Radley (ed.) *Worlds of Illness: biographical and cultural perspectives on health and disease.* Routledge, London, pp. 124–42.

Boyle M (1990) *Schizophrenia: a scientific delusion?* Routledge, London.

Bracken P and Thomas P (2001) Postpsychiatry: a new direction for mental health. *BMJ.* **322**(24 March): 724–7.

Britten N (1994) Patient demand for prescriptions: a view from the other side. *Family Practice.* **11**(1): 62–6.

Britten N (2004) Patients' expectations of consultations. *BMJ.* **328**(21 February): 416–17.

Burkitt Wright E, Holcombe C and Salmon P (2004) Doctors' communication of trust, care, and respect in breast cancer: qualitative study. *BMJ.* **328**(10 April): 864–7.

Bury M (1982) Chronic illness as biographical disruption. *Sociology of Health and Illness.* **4**: 167–82.

Bury M (2001) Illness narrative: fact or fiction? *Sociology of Health and Illness.* **23**(3): 263–85.

Butler CC and Evans M (1999) The 'heartsink' patient revisited. *British Journal of General Practice.* **49**: 230–3.

Callan A and Littlewood R (1988) Patient satisfaction: ethnic origin or explanatory model? *International Journal of Social Psychology.* **44**(1): 1–11.

Calnan M (1998) Towards a conceptual framework of lay evaluation of health care. *Social Science and Medicine.* **27**(9): 927–33.

Calnan M and Williams S (1996) Lay evaluation of scientific medicine and medical care. In: S Williams and M Calnan (eds) *Modern Medicine: lay perspectives and experience.* UCL Press, London, pp. 26–46.

Cape J (2001) How general practice patients with emotional problems presenting with somatic or psychological symptoms explain their improvement. *British Journal of General Practice.* **51**(470): 724–9.

Carr-Hill R, Jenkins-Clarke S, Dixon P and Pringle M (1998) Do minutes count? Consultation lengths in general practice. *Journal of Health Services Research and Policy.* **3**(4): 207–13.

Chetley A (1990) *A Healthy Business? World health and the pharmaceutical industry.* Zed Books, London.

Clark NM and Gong M (2000) Management of chronic disease by practitioners and patients: are we teaching the wrong things? *BMJ.* **320**: 572–5.

Cohen D, McCubbin M, Collin J and Perodeau G (2001) Medications as social phenomena. *Health.* **5**(4): 441–69.

Cornwell J (1985) *Hard Earned Lives: accounts of health and illness from East London*. Tavistock, London.

Cox K, Stevenson F, Britten N and Dundar Y (2004) *A Systematic Review of Communication Between Patients and Health Care Professionals About Medicine-taking and Prescribing*. Medicines Partnership, London.

Coyle J (1999) Exploring the meaning of 'dissatisfaction' with health care: the importance of 'personal identity threat'. *Sociology of Health and Illness*. **21**: 95–124.

Crawford MJ and Kessel AS (1999) Not listening to patients – the use and misuse of patient satisfaction studies. *International Journal of Social Psychiatry*. **45**(1): 1–7.

Department of Health (1999) *Patient and Public Involvement in the new NHS*. Department of Health, London.

Department of Health (2000) *The NHS Plan: a plan for investment, a plan for reform*. Department of Health, London.

Department of Health (2001) *Involving Patients and the Public in Healthcare: a discussion document*. Department of Health, London.

Department of Health (2003) *Building on the Best: choice, responsiveness and equity in the NHS*. Department of Health, London.

Department of Health (2005) *Delivering Choosing Health – Making Healthier Choices Easier*. Department of Health, London.

DHSS (1983) *NHS Management Inquiry (The Griffiths Management Report)*. DHSS, London.

Dieppe P, Bartlett C, Davey P, Doyal L and Ebrahim S (2004) Balancing benefits and harms: the example of non-steroidal anti-inflammatory drugs. *BMJ*. **329**(3 July): 31–4.

Dixon-Woods M and Critchley S (1999) Medical and lay views of irritable bowel syndrome. *Family Practice*. **17**(2): 108–13.

Donaldson L (2003) Expert patients usher in a new era of opportunity for the NHS. *BMJ*. **326**(14 June): 1279–80.

Donovan J and Blake D (2000) Qualitative study of interpretation of reassurance among patients attending rheumatology clinics: just a touch of arthritis, doctor?. *BMJ*. **320**: 541–4.

Edwards A, Elwyn G, Smith C, Williams S and Thornton H (2001) Consumers' views of quality in the consultation and their relevance to 'shared decision-making' approaches. *Health Expectations*. **4**(3): 151–61.

Edwards C, Staniszweska S and Crichton N (2004) Investigation of the ways in which patients' reports of their satisfaction with healthcare are constructed. *Sociology of Health and Illness*. **26**(2): 159–83.

Edwards T (1999) Drug interactions: deadly cocktails. *What Doctors Don't Tell You*. **10**(6): 1–3.

Eisenberg L (1978) Disease and illness: distinctions between professional and popular ideas of sickness. *Culture Medicine and Psychiatry*. **1**: 9–21.

Eisenberg L (1981) The physician as interpreter: ascribing meaning to the illness experience. *Comprehensive Psychiatry*. **22**(3): 239–48.

Elwyn G and Gwyn R (1999) Stories we hear and stories we tell: analysing talk in clinical practice. *BMJ*. **318**(16 January): 186–8.

Epstein RM (2000) Time, autonomy and satisfaction. *Journal of General Internal Medicine*. **15**: 517–18.

Evans-Pritchard EE (1937) *Witchcraft, Oracles and Magic Among the Azande*. Oxford University Press, Oxford.

Fitzgerald F (1994) The tyranny of health. *New England Journal of Medicine*. **331**(July 21): 196–8.

Frank A (1995) *The Wounded Storyteller: body, illness, and ethics*. University of Chicago Press, Chicago.

Frankel R and Beckman H (1989) Evaluating the patient's primary problem. In: M Stewart and DL Roter (eds) *Communicating with Medical Patients*. Sage Publications, London.

Gabe J and Bury M (1996) Anxious times: the benzodiazepine controversy and the fracturing of expert authority. In: P Davis (ed.) *Contested Ground: public purpose and private interest in the regulation of prescription drugs*. Oxford University Press, Oxford, pp. 42–56.

Galvin R (2002) Disturbing notions of chronic illness and individual responsibility: towards a genealogy of morals. *Health*. **6**(2): 107–37.

Gask L, Rogers A, Oliver D, May C and Roland M (2003) Qualitative study of patients' perceptions of the quality of care for depression in general practice. *British Journal of General Practice*. **53**: 278–83.

Gerrard TJ and Riddell JD (1988) Difficult patients: black holes and secrets. *BMJ*. **297**(20 August): 532–3.

Giacomini MK, Cook DJ, Streiner DL and Anand SS (2001) Guidelines as rationing tools: a qualitative analysis of psychosocial patient selection criteria for cardiac procedures. *Canadian Medical Association Journal*. **164**(5): 634.

Good B (1994) *Medicine, Rationality, and Experience: an anthropological perspective*. Cambridge University Press, Cambridge.

Groves JE (1978) Taking care of the hateful patient. *New England Journal of Medicine*. **298**(16): 883–7.

Harrison A and New B (2002) *Public Interest, Private Decisions: health-related research in the UK*. King's Fund, London.

Heath I (1998) Following the story: continuity of care in general practice. In: T Greenhalgh and B Hurwitz (eds) *Narrative Based Medicine: dialogue and discourse in clinical practice*. BMJ Books, London, pp. 83–92.

Heath I (2003) A wolf in sheep's clothing: a critical look at the ethics of drug taking. *BMJ*. **327**(11 October): 856–8.

Horne R and Weinman J (2004) The theoretical basis of concordance and issues for research. In: C Bond (ed.) *Concordance: a partnership in medicine taking*. Pharmaceutical Press, London, pp. 119–45.

Howie JGR, Heaney DJ, Maxwell M, Walker JJ, Freeman GK and Rai H (1999) Quality at general practice consultations: cross sectional survey. *BMJ*. **319**: 738–43.

Hyden, L-C (1997) Illness and narrative. *Sociology of Health and Illness*. **19**(1): 48–69.

Institute of Medicine (2000) *To Err is Human: building a safer health system*. National Academy Press, Washington DC. http://books.nap.edu/books/0309068371/html (accessed 28 September 2005).

Jackson JL, Chamberlin J and Kroenke K (2001) Predictors of patient satisfaction. *Social Science and Medicine*. **52**: 609–20.

Jacobsen B, Smith A and Whitehead M (1991) *The Nation's Health, A Strategy for the 1990s: a report from an independent multidisciplinary committee*. King Edward's Hospital Fund for London, London.

Kangas I (2001) Making sense of depression: perceptions of melancholia in lay narratives. *Health*. **5**(1): 76–92.

Kawachi I and Conrad P (1996) Medicalization and the pharmacological treatment of blood pressure. In: P Davis (ed.) *Contested Ground: public purpose and private interest in the regulation of prescription drugs*. Oxford University Press, Oxford, pp. 26–41.

Kelstrup A, Lund K, Lauritsen B and Bech P (1993) Satisfaction with care reported by psychiatric inpatients. Relationship to diagnosis and medical treatment. *Acta Psychiatrica Scandinavica*. **87**: 374–9.

Kettunen T, Poskiparta M, Liimatainen L, Sjogren A and Karhila P (2001) Taciturn patients in health counselling at a hospital: passive recipients or active participators? *Qualitative Health Research*. **11**(3): 399–410.

Kleinman A (1980) *Patients and Healers in the Context of Culture: an exploration of the borderland between anthropology, medicine and psychiatry*. University of California Press, Berkeley.

Kleinman A (1988) *The Illness Narratives: suffering, healing and the human condition*. Basic Books, United States.

Knight R (1987) The importance of list size and consultation length as factors in general practice. *Journal of the Royal College of General Practitioners.* **37**: 19–22.

Kutchins H and Kirk SA (1999) *Making us Crazy: DMS – the psychiatric bible and the creation of mental disorders.* Constable, London.

Launer J (2002) *Narrative-based Primary Care: a practical guide.* Radcliffe Medical Press, Oxford.

Launer J (2003) Narrative-based medicine: a passing fad or a giant leap for general practice? *British Journal of General Practice.* **Feb**: 91–2.

Letendre R (1997) The everyday experience of psychiatric hospitalization: the user's viewpoint. *International Journal of Social Psychiatry.* **43**: 285–98.

Ley P (1982) Satisfaction, compliance and communication. *British Journal of Clinical Psychology.* **21**: 241–54.

Lupton D (1997) Consumerism, reflexivity and the medical encounter. *Social Science and Medicine.* **45**(3): 373–81.

Martin CM, Banwell CL, Broom DH and Nisa M (1999) Consultation length and chronic illness care in general practice: a qualitative study. *Medical Journal of Australia.* **171**: 77–81.

Marvel MK, Epstein RM, Flowers K and Beckman HB (1999) Soliciting the patient's agenda: have we improved? *Journal of the American Medical Association.* **281**(3): 283–7.

May C, Gayle A, Chapple A, Chew-Graham CA, Dixon C, Gask L, Graham R, Rogers A and Roland M (2004) Framing the doctor–patient relationship in chronic illness: a comparative study of general practitioner's accounts. *Sociology of Health and Illness.* **26**(2): 135–58.

McIver S (1991) *An Introduction to Obtaining the Views of Users of Health Services.* King's Fund, London.

Medawar C (1997) The antidepressant web: marketing depression and making medicines work. *International Journal of Risk and Safety in Medicine.* **10**: 75–126.

Meredith P (1993) Patient satisfaction with communication in general surgery: problems of measurement and improvement. *Social Science and Medicine.* **37**(5): 591–602.

Misselbrook D (2001) *Thinking About Patients.* Petroc Press, Newbury.

Morrell DC, Evans ME, Morris RW and Roland MO (1986) The 'five minute' consultation: effect of time constraint on clinical content and patient satisfaction. *BMJ.* **292**: 870–3.

Morris DB (1998) *Illness and Culture in the Postmodern Age.* University of California Press, Berkeley.

Mulcahy L and Tritter JQ (1998) Pathways, pyramids and icebergs? Mapping the links between dissatisfaction and complaints. *Sociology of Health and Illness.* **20**(6): 825–47.

O'Dowd TC (1988) Five years of heartsink patients in general practice. *BMJ.* **297**(20 August): 530–2.

Ogden J, Bavalia K, Bull M, Frankum S, Goldie C, Gosslau M, Jones A, Kumar S and Vasant K (2004) 'I want more time with my doctor': a quantitative study of time and the consultation. *Family Practice.* **21**(5): 479–83.

Petit-Zeman S, Sandamas G and Hogman G (2001) *Doesn't It Make You Sick? Side effects of medicine and physical health concerns of people with severe mental illness.* NSF, London.

Pirmohamed M, James S, Meakin S, Green C, Scott AK, Walley TJ, Farrar K, Park BK and Breckenridge AM (2004) Adverse drug reactions as cause of admission to hospital: prospective analysis of 18 820 patients. *BMJ.* **329**(3 July): 15–19.

Pollock K and Grime J (2002) Patients' perceptions of entitlement to time in general practice consultations for depression: qualitative study. *BMJ.* **325**(28 September): 687.

Radley A (1993) The role of metaphor in adjustment to chronic illness. In: A Radley (ed.) *Worlds of Illness: biographical and cultural perspectives on health and disease.* Routledge, London, pp. 109–23.

Raine R, Carter S, Sensky T and Black N (2004) General practitioners' perceptions of chronic fatigue syndrome and beliefs about its management, compared with irritable bowel syndrome: qualitative study. *BMJ.* **328**: 1354–7.

Rees Lewis J (1994) Patient views on quality care in general practice: literature review. *Social Science and Medicine*. **39**(5): 655–70.

Richards H, Reid M and Watt G (2003) Victim-blaming revisited: a qualitative study of beliefs about illness causation, and responses to chest pain. *Family Practice*. **20**(6): 711–16.

Rogers A, Pilgrim D and Lacey R (1993) *Experiencing Psychiatry: a user's view of services*. Macmillan/MIND, Basingstoke.

Roland MO, Bartholomew J, Courteney MJF, Morris RW and Morrell DC (1986) The 'five minute' consultation: effect of time constraint on verbal communication. *BMJ*. **292**: 874–6.

Roth JA (1986) Some contingencies of the moral evaluation and control of clientele: the case of the hospital emergency service. In: P Conrad and R Kern (eds) *The Sociology of Health and Illness: critical perspectives* (2e). St Martin's Press, New York, pp. 322–33.

Salkeld G, Solomon M, Short L and Butow PN (2004) A matter of trust – patient's views on decision-making in colorectal cancer. *Health Expectations*. **7**: 104–14.

Shapiro J, Mosqueda L and Botros D (2003) A caring partnership: expectations of ageing persons with disabilities for their primary care doctors. *Family Practice*. **20**(6): 635–41.

Shaw J (2004) A policy framework for concordance. In: C Bond (ed.) *Concordance: a partnership in medicine taking*. Pharmaceutical Press, London, pp. 147–66.

Sinding C (2003) Disarmed complaints: unpacking satisfaction with end-of-life care. *Social Science and Medicine*. **57**: 1375–85.

Sitzia J and Wood N (1997) Patient satisfaction: a review of issues and concepts. *Social Science and Medicine*. **45**(12): 1829–43.

Stallard P (1996) The role and use of consumer satisfaction surveys in mental health services. *Journal of Mental Health*. **5**(4): 333–48.

Stimson G and Webb B (1975) *Going to See the Doctor: the consultation process in general practice*. Routledge and Kegan Paul, London.

Stricker BH and Psaty BM (2004) Detection, verification, and quantification of adverse drug reactions. *BMJ*. **329**(3 July): 44–7.

Strong P (1979) *The Ceremonial Order of the Clinic: patients, doctors and medical bureaucracies*. Routledge and Kegan Paul, London.

Sullivan M (2003) The new subjective medicine: taking the patient's point of view on health care and health. *Social Science and Medicine*. **56**(7): 1595–604.

Szasz TS (1970) *The Manufacture of Madness*. Harper and Row, New York.

Tate P (2003) *The Doctor's Communication Handbook* (4e). Radcliffe Medical Press, Oxford.

Towle A and Godolphin W (1999) Framework for teaching and learning informed shared decision making. *BMJ*. **319**(18 September): 766–71.

Townsend P, Davidson N and Whitehead M (1990) *Inequalities in Health: the Black Report and the health divide*. Penguin, Harmondsworth.

Townsend P, Phillimore P and Beattie A (1988) *Health and Deprivation: inequality and the North*. Routledge, London.

Tuckett D, Boulton M, Olson C and Williams A (1985) *Meetings Between Experts: an approach to sharing ideas in medical consultations*. Tavistock, London.

Vandenbrouke JP (2004) Benefits and harms of drug treatments. *BMJ*. **329**(3 July): 2–3.

Vuckovic N and Nichter M (1997) Changing patterns of pharmaceutical practice in the United States. *Social Science and Medicine*. **44**(9): 1285–302.

Werner A and Malterud K (2003) It is hard work behaving as a credible patient: encounters between women with chronic pain and their doctors. *Social Science and Medicine*. **57**: 1409–19.

West P (1976) The physician and the management of childhood epilepsy. In: M Wadsworth and D Robinson (eds) *Studies in Everyday Medical Life*. Martin Robertson, London.

White S (2002) Accomplishing 'the case' in paediatrics and child health: medicine and morality in inter-professional talk. *Sociology of Health and Illness*. **24**(4): 409–35.

Wiggers JH and Sanson-Fisher R (1997) Duration of general practice consultations:

association with patient occupational and educational status. *Social Science and Medicine*. **44**(7): 925–34.

Wilkinson R (1996) *Unhealthy Societies*. Routledge, London.

Williams B (1994) Patient satisfaction: a valid concept? *Social Science and Medicine*. **38**(4): 509–16.

Williams B, Coyle J and Healy D (1998) The meaning of patient satisfaction: an explanation of high reported levels. *Social Science and Medicine*. pp. 1351–9.

Williams B and Wilkinson G (1995) Patient satisfaction in mental health care. *British Journal of Psychiatry*. **166**: 559–62.

Williams G (1984) The genesis of chronic illness: narrative reconstruction. *Sociology of Health and Illness*. **6**: 175.

Williams M and Neal RD (1998) Time for a change? The process of lengthening booking intervals in general practice. *British Journal of General Practice*. **48**: 1783–6.

Williams S, Weinman J, Dale J and Newman S (1995) What do primary care patients want from their GP and how far does meeting expectations affect patient satisfaction? *Family Practice*. **12**: 193–201.

Wilson A (1991) Consultation length in general practice: a review. *British Journal of General Practice*. **41**: 119–22.

Chapter Ten

Conclusion

The concept of concordance in medical consultations has developed from a concern with patient non-compliance and the desire to reduce it (RPSGB 1997). In its original formulation, although incorporating a particular focus on medicines, concordance was viewed as an integral aspect of care, rather than a discrete or narrow component. A novel element was its acknowledgement of the patient perspective, and recognition of the primacy of patient preferences in negotiated decisions about treatment. Concordance referred to the *relationship* between patient and health professional, and thus to the entire consultation in which this was expressed. Attention was refocused from a preoccupation with non-compliance as a technical problem to the realisation that a radical shift in the underlying philosophy and culture of medical practice was required. The consultation was formulated as a dialogue between patient and professional. The professional had much to learn and benefit from this exchange, particularly an increased understanding of the patient's experience of illness and the values and aspirations underpinning his preferences for treatment. Prescribing could not be detached from the relationship between doctor and patient, or health behaviour from the rest of life.

Several trends have worked to support the ideology of concordance in the modern context of high levels of chronic (and expensive) illness among the ageing populations of modern industrial societies. Many people have to live with the long-term consequences of illness and disability. A choice of treatment is often available, and the benefits of treatment may be uncertain or marginal. In such circumstances, it is increasingly seen to be up to the individual to assume at least some responsibility for decision making in accordance with his personal outcome goals and tolerance of risk. Contemporary notions of citizenship accord priority to an individual autonomy and self-determination which is expressed directly in the exercise of choice: the role of patient is reconstituted as that of reflexive consumer. Concordance also fits well with the current policy focus on patient-centred medicine. This is promoted as a means of improving the quality of care through responsiveness to patient preference and assessment. It is also assumed to be a means to the delivery of more efficient, accountable and cost-effective services.

Although very much in tune with modern trends and policy preoccupations, the concept of concordance can also be linked to a longstanding critique of biomedicine. The professional preoccupation with non-compliance is understood as an ideological construct and manifestation of professional dominance riding on the success of biomedicine through to the middle decades of the twentieth century (*see* Chapter 2). This ideology privileges medical knowledge and professional authority over lay understanding and patients' experience of illness. The patient defect model is born out of professional assumptions about lay ignorance and incompetence. Attempted solutions to the problem of non-compliance have focused on attempts to manipulate patient behaviour, largely through the unidirectional transfer of technical information. The professional focus on patient education persists despite considerable evidence that more information does not make people more likely to take their medicines.

Compliance was justified by scientific authority and professional competence. Early research in this area recognised the ethical imperative of providing well informed patients with accurate diagnoses and safe and effective treatment in return for their obedience to medical prescription. As the ideology of compliance has been appropriated as a tool for maintaining professional dominance, the patient deficit model has come to eclipse this awareness of professional obligation. In recent decades, however, things have got more difficult. Alongside modern notions of citizenship which stress personal autonomy and freedom of choice, and a policy orientation to increased professional accountability, biomedicine has been subject to a series of sustained critiques since the middle decades of the last century. At the same time as the rising burden of chronic illness exposes its therapeutic limitations, biomedicine's technological prowess reveals an awesome capacity to harm: iatrogenic illness has become a substantial cause of morbidity and death. To make matters worse, evidence of the variable and inconsistent nature of professional practice has called in question the extent to which medicine is truly 'scientific' and undermines the basis of its privilege and authority. Evidence-based medicine has developed as an influential movement which aims to purge the idiosyncracies of clinical judgement through the dissemination of canons of best practice based on the development of a sound and authoritative evidence base (*see* Chapter 3).

Evidence-based medicine is seen by its proponents as a way of reclaiming the high ground and restoring the scientific authority of medicine. However, its positivist perspective is directly opposed to the principles of patient-centred medicine, which prioritise the patient's subjective experience of illness and require a professional sensitivity to patient values and preferences which may conflict with the dictates of clinical rationality. Sociological analysis from the 1970s onwards began to reveal the complexity of lay concepts of health and illness and also the extent to which people assumed responsibility themselves for the day-to-day management of their health and illness (*see* Chapter 4). This work shed new light on health behaviours, including medicine taking, and demonstrated the importance of the social and personal significance of ideas and beliefs in determining such behaviour. In particular, a large body of literature has established a widespread dislike of taking medicines throughout the population. Medicines may be valued as a means of restoring or maintaining normal function and social and economic participation, but resisted as unwelcome signifiers of illness and dependency. Non-compliance is a manifestation of such resistance, and often the result of reasoned experiments that patients conduct to test out the efficacy or need for medicines

In contrast to the active management of their health and the critical scrutiny that people bring to bear on professional judgement from outside the consultation, a great deal of evidence testifies to the passive deference of patients in the course of their encounters with professionals (*see* Chapter 5). The durability of the traditional patient role and the stylised bureaucratic format of medical consultations in the face of prolonged and substantial pressures for change is perplexing. Nevertheless, decades of exhortations for professionals to improve their communication skills and become attuned to a more holistic and patient-centred practice, and for patients to take a more active, informed and participatory role in the consultation have gone mostly little more than skin-deep. Professional authority has resisted sustained pressure for change from many sources – policy goals for increased accountability, the development of consumerism, critiques of biomedicine, iatrogenisis, professional dominance and medicalisation as well as the disenchantment with science and the grand narrative of technological mastery which characterises the world view of postmodern society. If anything, the pervasive influence of professional medicine has become woven more deeply into the fabric of everyday life. Its function as a self-regulatory mechanism of social control has spread, rather than contracted, with the growth of a 'coercive healthism' which perpetuates a political focus on the individual, rather than social, determinants of illness, and increasingly drives towards a linkage between conformist and self-disciplined behaviour and entitlement to healthcare.

Patient-centred medicine and genuine patient involvement in healthcare remain rare. The medical consultation continues to be an arena in which even the most informed and articulate consumers 'dumb down', adopting a passive and deferential stance in relation to professionals with whom they do not necessarily agree, but on whose services and goodwill they depend. The etiquette of the consultation has evolved as a way of containing the intrinsic difficulties of the occasion as potentially highly threatening to the face of both patient and professional (*see* Chapter 6). Both parties routinely strive to avoid the expression of conflict and tension that could jeopardise the immediate encounter and damage relationships in the longer term. The idealisation of professional expertise and lay ignorance renders patients' active questioning liable to be construed as threatening and challenging behaviour, and thus to be avoided. Patient reticence and taciturnity tends to be interpreted as acceptance and understanding, inhibiting the development of a professional reflexivity that would enable a more sensitive awareness of the patient perspective and agenda. Detailed analysis of the interaction between patients and health professionals reveals the substantial contribution which patients make in observing the norms and etiquette of the consultation. However, its success as a social encounter is often achieved at the expense of its effectiveness as a therapeutic encounter. Professional status is reinforced by patient deference. Both parties cooperate in the enactment of their accustomed roles. The norms of social interaction produce barriers that are built into the organisation of the consultation and the structure of communication that constrains the realisation of concordance.

Although routine events for professionals, medical consultations are often difficult and emotionally charged encounters for patients. Concordance increases the challenge of the consultation for both parties, in opening up, perhaps even encouraging, the expression of disagreement and conflict that would normally remain hidden. The benefits of concordance are anticipated to be considerable, but it remains a risky strategy, which both patients and professionals may be reluctant to adopt. These communicative and organisational barriers to concordance go some way to accounting for the durability of the bureaucratic format of the consultation in the face of considerable social, policy and ideological pressures to change. The principles of concordance are also deeply challenging to professional roles and culture. Treatment goals and outcome evaluation come to be determined (subjectively) by the patient rather than the ('objective') criteria of clinical rationality (*see* Chapter 7). This strikes at the heart of professional exclusiveness and expertise. Indeed, a further stumbling block to concordance transcending aspiration is the widespread professional resistance to the idea of patient expertise. Apprehension, and often the assumption, that patients will make bad and damaging – not to mention expensive – decisions run like a leitmotif through the professional literature relating to shared decision making. The structured asymmetry of the consultation, in which the professional holds interactional dominance, stifles the scope for patient choice through techniques of framing and the selective presentation of information. The result is often merely 'pseudoconcordance', shielding the perpetuation of professional paternalism, or at best, 'informed compliance'.

Information is widely regarded as key to the development of patient-centred medicine and shared decision making (*see* Chapter 8). Control of specialist knowledge has been an important source of professional status and authority. The emergence of highly educated populations and an information revolution which places the most esoteric knowledge at the fingertips of anyone with access to a computer and internet connection have eroded this professional monopoly. They *should* be a powerful stimulus to increasing patient involvement in medical consultations and decision making and democratising relationships between patients and professionals. Good information is a prerequisite for the autonomy and self-determination which is a core attribute of modern citizenship. As the focus on individual responsibility for 'choosing' health intensifies, 'health literacy' is becoming an essential component of personal competence. There is, increasingly, an obligation to be informed.

Patient dissatisfaction with professional provision of information has been frequently reported. There is a good deal of evidence that information about medicines, in particular, is often inadequate. Patients' desire to be 'fully informed' is widely assumed to be nearly universal. The nature of what constitutes 'full' information tends to remain unspecified and unproblematic. However, it is becoming apparent that patients' preferences are far from uniform, and often varied and equivocal. The effects of knowledge are not always benign. The whole issue of how individuals process expert knowledge is complex and problematic, and its impact on their relationships with health professionals uncertain. Information may be reassuring, but also threatening; liberating, but also burdensome. It may enhance coping, but also increase anxiety, and augment rather than diminish uncertainty. Resisting information can also be a way of coping with illness. Equally, knowledge may be a means of resisting professional power and intervention. Knowledge cannot be taken back, or 'unknown', nor can its effects be anticipated in advance. It is often difficult to be aware of exactly what there is to know, or how much information is needed. More information does not necessarily lead to better decisions. Knowledge also implies responsibility, and it is evident that patients do not always want to assume an active role in making decisions about their healthcare. This is especially likely when they are confronted with momentous choices and serious ill health.

In the literature on patient-centred medicine and shared decision making illness makes a discrete appearance. Its portrayal is sanitised and idealised so that it is easy to get the impression that provided the 'right' decision is reached and patients are sufficiently well informed to understand why they need to follow medical prescription and advice, as well as how to do so, all will be well. The *experience* of illness as overwhelming, painful, miserable, frightening, enduring and terminal is overlooked. In reality, medical interventions are not always effective, and may cause harm. Often, the best they can provide is amelioration of symptoms and discomfort caused by chronic, degenerative conditions or prolongation of lives blighted by terminal disease. Diagnosis is frequently uncertain, and the best course of action is often unclear, even to experts. Non-specific and indeterminate functional disorders and psychosocial distress comprise a large component of the burden of morbidity. People seek to contain the disruption of illness, to reduce its significance and engage in lives that are fulfilling and, as far as possible, 'normal'. 'Getting on with life' may be accorded higher priority than the acquisition of expertise in technical aspects of treatment that are considered more appropriately left to professionals. Indeed, the considerable investment of time and effort involved in becoming a quasi expert in such areas may be regarded as simply burdensome and unnecessary.

Giddens (1991) has depicted the complex, abstract systems of expertise on which citizens of modern societies depend for the management of their everyday life and affairs as a source of pervasive unease. A sense of indeterminacy derives from the lack of individual (or even collective) control and because the consequences of organisational malfunction or failure may be catastrophic. Nevertheless, within the realm of everyday experience, the operation of such systems delivers considerable and usually reliable benefits, conferring an unprecedented degree of personal security and opportunity. The need to rely on expert systems which are beyond personal control generates one of the basic tensions of modern living. However, the complexity of such systems places them *practically* beyond the reach of all but specialists. It is not possible to acquire expertise in more than a few small areas over the course of an individual lifetime. People may be willing to assume greater personal involvement in matters relating to health and illness than other areas of their life and affairs, such as banking or computer maintenance. This is more likely to happen if they confront the need to manage serious or long-term illness, and particularly if they feel their trust has been abused, or the expert system has in some way failed them. Increased awareness of conflicting and inconsistent knowledge even within, as well as between, expert systems of knowledge and their practitioners is another of the tensions to be confronted in modern life. However, this does not mean that under ordinary circumstances most people feel that it is necessary, or even appropriate, to try to turn themselves into quasi-professionals.

It is striking that both doctors and patients still regard doctors to be the most important source of information about illness and treatment. Whatever the *potential* impact of the internet and other media of information transfer, it is easy to overstate its influence to date. It is certainly evident that patients do not consider written or textual information as a substitute for verbal communication with professionals. Patients value different kinds of information and often privilege experience over technical expertise in the effort to construct a coherent explanation and understanding of arbitrary and inexplicable events and experiences (the 'effort after meaning'). An important reason for valuing verbal information rather than written is the opportunity it presents for patients to build relationships with professionals and for professionals to demonstrate their respect for patients, who strive to be recognised as individuals rather than cases.

Information does not substitute for empathy. Perhaps even more than wanting to be informed, patients desire to feel that they have been acknowledged and understood. Indeed, Kleinman (1988) proposes that for the substantial proportion of patients confronted by the exigencies of chronic, terminal or functional disorders, and for whom effective therapies are either limited or exhausted, the provision of compassionate support and understanding ('empathic witnessing') may be the most that health professionals have to offer (*see* Chapter 9).

It is not so much the information that is conveyed as the understanding that is negotiated that is important in determining patient 'satisfaction' and the success of the consultation. Conflict and disparity between lay and professional models of pathology are frequent sources of dissatisfaction and disappointment. *Effective* communication bridges the gap between these. Considerable interest has been focused on the role of illness narratives in making sense of illness and attempting to repair the disruption of life. Such narratives reveal the reality of the struggle and challenge of illness, as people strive to cope with the practical and existential problems it poses. The bureaucratic format of the consultation inhibits patients' ability to tell their stories, and the biomedical worldview overlooks their significance, directing attention to the objective manifestations of disease, rather than the subjective experience of illness.

It is difficult for patient narratives to displace the professional narratives which may pathologise, rather than reconstruct, their experience, e.g. in terms of pejorative labels such as 'fibromyalgia', or 'depression', and negative attributions of 'difficult' or 'demanding' patients. These override the significance of patient narratives as a pedagogical resource and source of professional insight. While patient narratives seek to account for and absorb the arbitrariness of illness, prevalent professional and policy narratives linking health and lifestyle increasingly present illness as fundamentally a matter of choice and personal control. Current ideologies of the autonomous self are manipulated into convenient propaganda, in which illness becomes predominantly an individual responsibility, rather than a social concern. Health is coming to be viewed as a basic competence, and attributions of blame and personal responsibility linked to entitlement to care.

Formal encouragement of increased personal responsibility for health and illness is expressed in the enthusiastic espousal of 'self-management programmes' and a more general commitment to the 'expert patient'. It remains an empirical question – and an important topic for investigation – how far patients are comfortable with the extended responsibilities of the 'expert patient' role. To the extent that it seeks to train patients to accept and self-manage their illness in line with conventional clinical judgements and practice, the Expert Patient initiative can be viewed as a further instance of professional incorporation rather than transformation and as an adaptive strategy of an established professional practice, in absorbing the pressure to change. The goals of 'self-management' are very different from the well established commitment to 'self-help', which has often developed in opposition to, and as a means of remedying the limitations and shortfall of professional provision. Concerns have also been voiced about the extent to which the extension of patient responsibility for the genesis and management of illness may be used to provide a convenient foil for the contraction of professional responsibility.

The reality of modern life is that individuals have to deal with large amounts of information. The skills required for doing this are becoming a basic requirement for personal achievement and social participation. Awareness of the shifting, conflicting and contested nature of 'knowledge' contributes to a sense of uncertainty and doubt among the citizens of late modern societies. The notion of the patient as reflexive consumer within a patient-centred system of healthcare reconfigures the traditional roles of patient and professional, and adds to the increasingly complex interrelations between these. It may be the trend towards increased patient responsibility and self-management of illness proves to be inexorable. However, the evidence to date indicates that there has been surprisingly little change in the form of the consultation, or the substance of the relationships between patients and healthcare professionals. I have suggested that this results partly from the inertia of a system which has evolved as an adaptive mechanism to contain the difficulties and tensions which are intrinsic features of the medical consultation as a social encounter. In addition, however, within the rhetoric of commitment to patient choice and patient-centred medicine are concealed a number of conflicting policies and trends which work against the realisation of concordance rather than towards it. The current preoccupation with evidence-based medicine and standardised guidelines and performance targets conflicts with the exercise of patient choice and clinical judgement which deviates from predefined norms. The sheer complexity of modern health systems make the transmission of meaning and shared understandings hard to carry through a network of communication. Wider concerns of organisational and professional hierarchy, and of interprofessional allegiance and collusion, work against full disclosure of information to patients and open discussion between patients and professionals. Professional medicine has been remarkably successful in adapting to change through a process of incorporation and assimilation, rather than a transformation of its practice (as in the formulation of the Expert Patient programme). In the end, however, a major brake on radical change within the system has been due to the conservative response of many patients.

The move to patient-centred medicine has been driven largely by policy makers on the one hand, and research academics on the other. It is the expression of a complex mix of motives and aspirations. These include the desire to reduce costs, to improve the quality of care, and a commitment to a view of modern citizenship which stresses the core attributes of autonomy and self-determination and views the paternalism of traditional medicine as ineffective and intolerable. While a significant minority of patients may espouse these ideals, the available evidence suggests that most are not yet comfortable with the role of reflexive consumer in relation to healthcare. Concepts of patient-centred medicine, shared decision making, satisfaction with healthcare and even concordance are professional (ideological) constructs, and their relevance to patients remains to be established. The ideals of concordance may be exemplary, but it is not yet clear to what extent they resonate with patient goals and concerns, and the desire to avoid, rather than engage with, conflict in the consultation. A bewildering array of research evidence has produced complex and varied results about the patient response to greater information and involvement in illness management, and the desire to share decisions with their doctors. However, several very consistent themes emerge about what patients search for in their quest for therapy: good relationships with professionals, reassurance, the feeling that their problems have been acknowledged and understood, and that they have been dealt with and valued as a person rather than a case. Overall, patients prefer to be heard, rather than instructed. Notwithstanding the sustained critique to which biomedicine has been subject for over half a century, the willingness of patients to place their trust in individual practitioners is striking. The tension between trust and knowledge requires further empirical investigation. However, it seems that within the normative rules of the medical encounter, neither patient nor professional is comfortable with the overt demonstration of patient expertise. In the ordinary course of events it seems also that many, perhaps even most, patients do not consider it appropriate or necessary to turn themselves into subject specialists about their own disease. People seek to be acquire *enough* information about illness, and to be *appropriately* involved in matters relating to their care and treatment. The variability of individual preferences and reactions makes the task of sensitively tailoring professional responses quite formidable. However, the quality of the relationship between patients and their doctors is a critical determinant of 'adequacy' in this context.

I am not trying to argue against the desirability of patients being provided with ready access to as much information as they require, or to be as fully involved in making decisions about illness management and treatment as they desire. I am emphatically not supporting the continuation of professional dominance and paternalism. The point is rather that the ideologically motivated commitment to patient choice and autonomy has run substantially ahead of the roles that most patients themselves feel comfortable with. Policy is framed in terms of assumptions about what patients want or regard as intrinsically desirable but which are not borne out by a careful review of the available evidence. In the preceding discussion, I have sought to establish that patient preferences for information and involvement in medical decision making and the determinants of their satisfaction with healthcare are much more variable and complex than is widely assumed, and require extensive further investigation. In particular, a greater knowledge and awareness of the organisational and interactional constraints which impinge on the practice of medicine and constrain the relationships between patients and health workers is required to develop a better understanding of how to effect a genuine change in professional culture and practice.

Where does this leave concordance? The promise of concordance lay in its potential to open up professional awareness of the nature of the patient perspective, and the importance of addressing this directly, through its incorporation into mainstream policy agenda. Patients and professionals who engage in more open and productive consultations are supposed to be more committed to treatment options they have played a part in selecting, and so the prescribing of inappropriate and wasted drugs and unwanted treatments should be substantially reduced. A great advantage of concordance over other models of shared decision making is that it accommodates a wide range of patient preferences and emphasises the diversity of negotiated outcomes. It also acknowledges the reality of conflict and dissent between patients and professionals, and even that it may not be possible to achieve consensus. The real goal of concordant consultations is that all parties *exchange* information, and share different perspectives as the basis of an increased understanding. Thus it is primarily focused on the relationship between patients and professionals rather than a specific outcome of the consultation. To this extent, the ideal of concordance held promise as a real contender in engineering a shift in professional culture and practice to bring it more in line with a genuinely patient-centred medicine (i.e. one that starts from patients' expressed concerns and preferences regarding their medical care).

In its original formulation concordance recognised the significance of the patient perspective and incorporated a focus on the process as well as the outcome of healthcare. It encouraged an acknowledgement of the *difficulty* of conducting successful consultations, and invited all participants to acknowledge the uncertainties and limitations of medical knowledge and treatment. This imposes greater demands on patients as well as professionals, and increases the challenge of an already difficult encounter. Given the rarity of concordance in practice, it is not yet possible to say whether the benefits of such encounters outweigh the costs. Realistically, the routinisation of concordance in all everyday medical consultations is an unlikely prospect. However, as a model or guide for such encounters and aspirational statement for the development of professional culture, it still holds value. In practice, however, the message of concordance has been distorted through its routine misapplication as a synonym for compliance. A slightly more sophisticated version of concordance is represented in the new orthodoxy in which it features as an instrument for increasing compliance (informed compliance). The lay perspective is taken on board in order to tailor information and explanation more sensitively to the goal of overriding patient misconceptions. Once the patient is able to *understand* the professional point of view, the barriers to compliance are assumed to crumble. Education is an entitlement supporting patient empowerment and enabling the active choice of health. Effectively, information is viewed as a means of training consumers to become better (more compliant) patients. Far from expressing an underlying philosophy of care, concordance has become reduced to a technique of patient persuasion. The goal of the consultation remains the substitution, rather than the translation, of different kinds of knowledge. The purpose, and the practice, of the professional is enhanced, rather than altered.

A truly patient-centred, and concordant, practice would start from an acknowledgement of the unpleasantness and *difficulty* posed by illness, and a greater knowledge of patients' experience and preferences regarding healthcare. Evidence from the preceding discussion suggests that this is likely to be more strongly oriented to understanding and empathy than information and autonomy. Heaping information about medicines onto patients is not sufficient to extend partnership, or achieve concordance. What really would 'empower' patients is the ability to define their needs and take a full part in the interprofessional discussion of their case. It is clear, for example, that services driven by mental health service users would result in a radical redistribution of resources, reduced emphasis on drugs and contraction of the role and influence of professional psychiatry. Psychological therapies would be greatly extended along with an increased provision of alternative recreational and occupational therapies. A service user centred system of healthcare would be oriented to a social rather than a biomedical model of mental health and illness. The emphasis would be on maintaining or restoring social and economic function and dealing constructively with personal and social adversity. While some positive initiatives have been undertaken in this direction, they are very far from mainstream.

The incorporation of concordance as an instrument for promoting compliance provides a good example of professional medicine's ability to absorb rather than respond to change, and so to protect its social status and authority. It represents a lost opportunity to promote the development of a more humane and patient-oriented medical practice, and to develop professional awareness of the problematic nature of medicines and medicine taking for many patients. This could, in turn, have opened up a wider debate about the social and personal significance of medicines. The preceding discussion has considered a considerable amount of evidence that current health policy is driven by professional and ideological assumptions, rather than an adequate knowledge of patients' experience of illness and preferences for healthcare. Issues around the implementation of patient partnership, information, shared decision making and concordance are much more complex and equivocal than they are commonly portrayed. The evidence considered in the preceding discussion has demonstrated how much still remains to be known about the lay perspective, from which a genuinely patient-centred medical practice could one day be developed.

References

Giddens A (1991) *Modernity and Self-Identity: self and society in the late modern age*. Polity Press, Oxford.

Kleinman A (1988) *The Illness Narratives: suffering, healing and the human condition*. Basic Books, United States.

RPSGB (1997) *From Compliance to Concordance: achieving shared goals in medicine taking*. London.

Index